I0695541

Health for the Whole Self

By: Cathy Duesterhoeft

Health for the Whole Self

Wellness is a state of being, which is different for everyone. It is achieved as each person reaches a healthy balance of a combination of things, including one's physical, emotional, spiritual, vocational, intellectual, and social health. In today's world of technology, you could access information on wellness with the touch of a computer key but that could be overwhelming as there is a wealth of information out there. I have made it easy for you by designing a daily dose of information that will help you on your path to wellness in small, easily digested pieces. Choose one of the daily suggestions and focus your attention on that one area, you won't be overwhelmed, and you won't be stressed; therefore, you are on your way to wellness one day at a time.

I have combined humor, ideas for physical fitness, nutrition information as well as quotes and study findings to make health and wellness a part of your new lifestyle. No more diets, no more quick fixes; just a new lifestyle of nutritious food and activity. Wellness is not so much a goal as a process, a journey, a way of orienting yourself toward life. It's a feeling of total participation that involves being in balance in the three key dimensions of body, mind, and spirit. These dimensions are always engaged in a dance. There is no separation between them.

Achieving emotional wellness is the ability to accept life's ups and downs. Health conditions, ranging from hives to cancer, may have as their origin, a breakdown in the body's immune system caused by the body's response to emotional stressors. Surrounding yourself with positive people, having a sense of humor and focusing on the positive are ways to improve this area of wellness.

The CDC reports that more than 65% of adult Americans are overweight and worse still, about a third of the adult population is obese. How did society get this way? During the 20th century, Western medicine and modern lifestyles have brought the populations of developed nations into high-risk status. I have given you examples of complementary and alternative medicine (CAM) and discussed the benefits of various physical activities, all to help you reach your wellness goals.

Spirituality is believing in a source of value that transcends the boundaries of the self but also nurtures the self. Spiritual wellness includes developing a strong sense of values, ethics, and morals. Spirituality is the way you find meaning, hope, comfort, and inner peace in your life. Many people find spirituality through religion. Some find it through music, art, or a connection with nature. You will find I have included scripture and quotes to help you find spiritual wellness.

You have the power to improve your life, and there's no better time than now to turn your potential into a reality. The health you deserve and the lifestyle you've always wanted are well within your reach.

Remember, break it down into small pieces so it's not overwhelming.

January 1:

Mind-

To avoid a feeling of failure, aim for the 90% solution. In any given day you have 10% of your time to feel angry, mad, sad, lonely, etc. You can spend this 10% arguing or crying but once your 10% is up, focus on the good.

Body-

If you got off track during the holidays, it's time to get back to a routine. Running will not only help shed new found pounds, but it will fight winter blues by clearing excess cortical. Regulating this hormone by lacing up will stabilize motivation, boost energy, and help you focus.

Spirit-

I can do everything through him who gives me strength. Philippians 4:13 (NIV)

January 2:

Mind-

A miracle is more than meets the eye. Whether it is divine intervention or a wonderful but unexpected occurrence, a miracle is beneficial and always welcomed.

Body-

Vinegar will slow the absorption of carbohydrates and prevent sudden surges in your blood sugar. It also slows the passage of food through your stomach, keeping you fuller for longer. Add some zest to pasta or potatoes with sun-dried tomato vinaigrette.

Spirit-

And whatever you do, whether in word or deed, do it all in the name of the Lord Jesus, giving thanks to God the Father through him.

Colossians 3:17

January 3:

Mind-

Make it a good day! Go out of your way to do something nice for a person in order to put a smile on your face as well as theirs.

Body-

Nine out of ten Americans aren't getting essential nutrients we need. Just one more serving of nutrient-rich milk per day can help fill the gap.

Spirit-

God adopts each of us into a family built on love. Call a family member you haven't spoken to in a while to make a connection.

January 4:

Mind-

Laugh often, love much! Whatever your day brings, enjoy it!

Body-

Diets are temporary…a lifestyle is permanent! By making small changes you are on track for a lifetime of wellness.

Spirit-

Life comes at us fast, but with God's help we can be ready.

January 5:

Mind-

"To find a friend one must close one eye. To keep him…two."
- Norman Douglas, author

Body-

Vegetables and fruits highest in potassium include spinach and other cooked greens, winter squash, white and sweet potatoes, tomato juice and sauce, bananas, citrus fruits, cantaloupe, dried apricots and raisins. By eating potassium rich foods, a person can reduce the risk of hypertension.

Spirit-

By dying for us, Christ affirmed that each of us is infinitely valuable.

January 6:

Mind-

What fills the heart shows in the face. If your heart is happy, your face will show it through a smile.

Body-

Taking a twenty- or thirty-minute run will help you organize your thoughts, clear your head, wake up, and return to your tasks with a clarity and energy that you can't get from coffee or even a nap.

Spirit-

What empty activity keeps me from spending time with God? Simplify your life to make time for prayer.

January 7:

Mind-

What are you focusing on today? Make it a goal to focus on positive thoughts in order to look at life through positive eyes.

Body-

Inactive people have a 90% greater risk of developing coronary heart disease than those who are physically active. Implement a simple walking plan to avoid heart disease. You do not need to walk far or fast to start feeling the effects. Once you start, make it a goal to increase your distance and speed a little at a time.

Spirit-

Praying can release us from anger and lead us toward peace. Asking for forgiveness is a freeing feeling.

January 8:

Mind-

When you are passionate about something it is easier to stick to it. Exercise should not be grueling. Pick something you like to do so you will be more willing to continue.

Body-

The most beneficial time for stretching comes at the end of doing anaerobic or resistance training workout. During this time muscles are thoroughly warmed up and can stretch maximally, but to a point of feeling mild tension with no discomfort.

Spirit-

When we look and listen, we will see and hear God. By taking time to sit quietly, a person can reduce stress and experience a sense of relaxation.

January 9:

Mind-

A laugh is a smile that bursts. Humor lightens your burden and brings your mind and body back into balance.

Body-

Yoga is a great exercise for overall mind and body fitness. It can help build your strength, lengthen your muscles, and help soothe stress. For beginners, a hatha class is the most appropriate style of yoga. Hatha is a slow-paced stretching class with some simple breathing exercises.

Spirit-

God invites us to pour out our heart in prayer. You do not need to use fancy words to pray, just speak from your heart. Tell God what is sitting heavy on your heart today.

January 10:

Mind-

Live each moment out loud. Shout for joy, laugh out loud, and share your excitement with those around you.

Body-

Polyphenols are antioxidant plant chemicals that may protect your body from cell and tissue damage linked to heart disease and certain cancers. Researchers found that among snack foods, popcorn has the highest polyphenol level. Air popped popcorn that is slightly salted is the healthiest type of popcorn to enjoy.

Spirit-

Life in Christ releases us from the past. Your past serves as an important guiding light, showing

you what can be done and what cannot. The
past cannot be changed.

January 11:

Mind-

Never stop exploring. Challenge yourself to learn
a new skill such as using a computer or knitting
to prevent winter blues from setting in.

Body-

Lying down within three or four hours of
consuming a large meal, particularly a late
dinner, could cause heartburn.

Spirit-

Go to God first. Do not try to figure out a
problem alone, ask God for help.

January 12:

Mind-

Achieve your dreams! If you have a deep desire to achieve a specific goal identify a path you can follow to accomplish that goal in order to achieve self-satisfaction.

Body-

In a recent study, researchers found that women with mild obesity (a body mass index of thirty) had a 35 percent greater risk of headaches that those with a lower BMI. Severe obesity (BMI of forty) upped the chances to 80 percent.

Spirit-

God calls us to go where we might never go on our own.

January 13:

Mind-

If you want to feel special, you have to *be* special. Everyone likes to feel special. Making your friends feel special is a great way to let them know how much you care about them. It takes some effort but after a short while it will come naturally to you. Making others feel special is a selfless act that can bring rays of sunshine into the lives of everyone around you.

Body-

Sprinkle one-fourth teaspoon of antioxidant-rich ground cinnamon on your morning oatmeal to perk up your day.

Spirit-

"Jesus said unto him, if thou canst believe, all things [are] possible to him that believeth."
~Mark 9:23

January 14:

Mind-

A smile can happen in a flash, but the memory can last a lifetime. Capture a memorable moment by taking a picture. Each time you look at that picture remember the fun you were having at the time.

Body-

When buying cereal, skip brands that have sugar listed as the first or second ingredient. Those products contain too much sweetener to be healthy.

Spirit-

God accepts me and declares me beloved. When you are feeling depressed remember that God

loves you at all times and will never abandon
you in your time of need.

January 15:

Mind-

Don't be so open minded that your brains fall
out. Funky colored hair, tattoos and piercings
seem to be the norm today. Expressing your true
self is important but you need to ask yourself,
"What does the Human Resource Director see
when she looks at me?" It will be hard to find a
job if you express yourself too fully.

Body-

Four steps to help you prevent cancer!

*Do not use tobacco products.
*Maintain a healthy weight throughout your life.
*Be physically active for thirty minutes or more
at least five days a week.

*Eat more vegetables, fruits, and whole grains and less red and processed meat.

Spirit-

"What good is it, my brothers, if a man claims to have faith but has no deeds? Can such faith save him?" James 2:14

January 16:

Mind-

Risk is the price you pay for opportunity. Risk can hold tremendous opportunities for those who know how to manage it but those who can't stomach risk are guaranteed to miss out on opportunities.

Body-

Sign up for a Zumba class. Zumba uses Latin music combined with easy dance moves to create a workout that can burn about six hundred to one thousand calories in an hour-long class.

Spirit-

This world's greatest thrills are nothing compared to being in God's presence. In all you do, make God your partner. Bring him along everywhere you go, talk to him throughout the day like you would a true friend.

January 17:

Mind-

Show up for life! You have one life to live so you need to enjoy it. Embrace opportunities that come your way and go looking for other opportunities like a class or new hobby. Just enjoy!

Body-

Leading a healthy lifestyle starts with the food you eat. Make it your goal to start each day with a healthy breakfast such as a whole grain bagel with low-fat cream cheese, an orange, and fat-free or low-fat milk.

Spirit-

Only by His grace! Life isn't always easy but if you have God in your life, you have a built-in support system. Think of Him as your private cheerleader.

January 18:

Mind-

" Talk low, talk slow, and don't say too much."
- John Wayne

Body-

While alcohol makes you sleepy, drinking it too close to bedtime can skew brain patterns, delay dream sleep and wake you up frequently during the night. Dinner is the ideal time to have a glass of wine because it gives your body enough time to metabolize the alcohol before you crawl into bed and start your sleep cycle.

Spirit-

If you look back over your life, you will see that you never grow during easy times; you grow during hard times. Working through hardship makes us stronger.

January 19:

Mind-

Make history; say thank you. Saying thank you seems so easy, but it is often the easiest thing that is forgotten. Make it a point to tell someone thank you today and watch how it brightens their face as well as your own.

Body-

Tickle the roof of your mouth to stop hiccups. Use a cotton ball to tickle the roof of your mouth at the point where the hard and soft palate meets. Hiccups are caused by a spasm of the diaphragm so tickling the roof of your mouth stimulates the vagus nerve, which interrupts that spasm.

Spirit-

"But to do good and to communicate forget not: for with such sacrifices God is well pleased. ~Hebrews 13:16

January 20:

Mind-

You can't paint by number all your life. Do you remember doing a paint by number art project when you were growing up? They can be fun but very restrictive in the sense that it doesn't allow for creativity. Do something creative today using paint but forget about the numbers.

Body-

Antioxidants help improve blood flow, which can help muscles contract more efficiently. Make a fruit salad using cantaloupe, peaches, and apricots to improve your blood flow.

Spirit-

Quiet time with God helps us to see what is truly important. Find ten or fifteen minutes in your day, sit in a comfortable chair, clear your mind of clutter, and focus on what God places on your heart.

January 21:

Mind-

"Go confidently in the direction of your dreams! Live the life you've imagined."

~ Henry David Thoreau

Body-

Feeling fatigued or confused? Get your brain back on track with fatty, omega-three rich fish like mackerel, trout, herring, tuna, and salmon. Match your lunch of fish with a salad of mixed greens to benefit your health even more.

Spirit-

In what ways do I reflect Christ in my life? As you go about your everyday errands today go out of your way to open the door for someone or allow someone to go in front of you at the checkout counter. Find a way to be Christlike and see the appreciation your attention gives the receiver.

January 22:

Mind-

Life is good! Focus on the positive today. Is there a snowstorm in the forecast? Look for the silver lining by using a day of vacation. Stay home and enjoy a good book and a cup oof hot chocolate made with low-fat milk.

Body-

Running releases more than just sweat. Exercise of any sort releases endorphins in the brain giving you a sense of euphoria. Try it out today by going for a brisk walk or an easy jog.

Spirit-

When our lives "shine for Jesus", others will notice. Other people notice when you are in a bad mood, but they also notice when you are in a good mood and feel happy. Share the happiness you feel from God's love with someone else.

January 23:

Mind-

Share your wisdom. Share what you have learned while traveling life's journey. Perhaps your wisdom can spare someone pain and heartache.

Body-

One cup of spinach contains approximately forty calories, while a cup of broccoli has 55 calories

and satisfies 20 percent of your day's fiber requirement. Most leafy greens are also a good source of calcium, an essential ingredient for muscle contraction.

Spirit-

Life is a song to sing and a place in the sun! Praise God through song today. It doesn't matter if you can't carry a tune. God does not care! Too bashful? Find a radio station that features Christian music and hum along.

January 24:

Mind-

Sometimes the key to happiness is appreciating the little things. Is it cold out today? Be thankful that you have a sweater or coat you can put on to keep warm. Remember, someone else always has it worse than you do.

Body-

Discomfort can be expected if you are challenging your body. However, if your exercise results in outright pain, it's probably excessive. Take it easy when you start out and build gradually to avoid injury.

Spirit-

The Lord rejoices when we mature spiritually. As you spend more time reading the bible, share what you read with someone else in order to spread His word.

January 25:

Mind-

Some relationships are meant to happen. Do you have a special friend that you can turn to when you need a shoulder to cry on? Why not honor that friend today by taking her to lunch at her favorite restaurant.

Body-

Shamans in the Amazon rain forest boiled the bark from the Brazil nut tree for a tea intended to detoxify the liver. A simple apple can provide the same benefit and is easier to find than bark from a Brazil nut tree.

Spirit-

We can be God's hands and feet for someone today. Find someone that needs assistance, whether it's grocery shopping, picking up mail or preparing a meal, your help will be appreciated.

January 26:

Mind-

Decide on one thing you want to accomplish this week and make a plan. Write down each step you need to carry out in order to accomplish your goal and enlist any help you may need.

Body-

For many years, baths and saunas have been popular methods of stimulating circulation and detoxifying the body in Finland, Germany and Sweden. You can experience the benefits of a hot bath right in your own home. Make your bath hot enough to induce a sweat. The process of perspiration removes toxins from the body.

Spirit-

Volunteering provides intangible benefits such as pride, satisfaction and accomplishment. To feel the satisfaction of service, ask yourself, "Who needs a helping hand from me today?"

January 27:

Mind-

It's always a good day when you wake up on the right side of the dirt. You have been given the gift of another day on God's earth so enjoy it to the fullest.

Body-

Run with and without music. Explore different routes. Try a new recipe. Switch classes at the gym. Changing your routine helps fight seasonal blahs and makes you a better- balanced athlete.

Spirit-

Walk in light and truth. Always strive to do the right thing. If you have knots in your stomach about something you said or did, chances are it was the wrong thing to say or do.

January 28:

Mind-

Try to learn more about someone you find annoying. By spending some time with them perhaps you will understand them a little better and come to overlook the part of them that annoys you.

Body-

Pears have especially high levels of a kind of fiber called pectin, which is known to help promote weight loss. Poached, they make a tasty warm dessert; raw, their creamy-gritty texture pairs nicely with cheese for a snack.

Spirit-

When we feel lost, knowing Scripture can create an internal map. When you feel lost and discouraged it is easy to forget that God is always with us, guiding us.

January 29:

Mind-

Discipline is necessary and character building. Gnawing and nagging is destructive. Make it your goal today to use discipline instead of punishment.

Body-

Tomatoes are high in fiber and have a high volume of water ensuring you get filled up with a minimum of calories. Plus, tomatoes increase in nutritional power when cooked. Blend up tomato soup-on a low-energy day, it is true comfort food.

Spirit-

Don't pile up empty yesterdays, get out there and live today. Get out there and live today. Live your life to the fullest. Pick one thing you always wanted to try and make it happen today.

January 30:

Mind-

Our development is an unfinished and ongoing story. We are always growing and learning; make sure your story has a happy ending.

Body-

Steaming spinach releases additional antioxidants. For extra flavor, add some garlic that's been chopped and left to stand for 10 minutes. The rest period allows the garlic to release a chemical called allicin that can help lower your risk of heart disease. For dinner tonight, match steamed spinach with a selection of lean protein.

Spirit-

Thank you, Jesus, for the amazing reality of your grace. Amen. There is no better role model than Jesus. He handled dying for our sins with grace and humility.

January 31:

Mind-

Life is a journey. It doesn't matter where your destination is. What matters is that you enjoy the experience of reaching that destination.

Body-

Muscular strength is best developed through high-intensity training. Lifting heavier loads, at a lower rep count until fatigue, tends to produce larger gains than lifting lighter loads many times to fatigue.

Spirit-

We can speak lovingly even when we disagree. When talking to someone, using a respectful tone is important. Talk to someone the way you would want to be talked to.

February 1:

Mind-

Winter isn't a favorite time of year for many folks-you can get cabin fever and the winter blues. Brighten your temperament, and your room with a coat of paint.

Body-

Purple potatoes have long been considered the food of gods. Seven thousand years ago they were reserved for Incan kings in their native Peru. Potatoes with the darkest colors have more than four times the antioxidant potential than other potatoes.

Spirit-

No matter where we wander, Christ seeks us. As a Christian you have a wonderful opportunity to share Christ's love with others. He is always with you and doesn't let you stray.

February 2:

Mind-

Peace for you is knowing that the simple things never change, and that life's filled with smiles to share and lessons to be learned, if we're only willing to listen. That's reminiscing.

Body-

When you consume plenty of fiber, it helps "clean" your intestines so that other nutrients, including vitamins and minerals, are better absorbed. Fiber also reduces the impact that sugars have on insulin levels and can lower cholesterol. A piece of fresh fruit for dessert is a great source of fiber.

Spirit-

Your life, energy, and love echo energetically to the very edges of all creation. You have that much energy. When your life is in balance there is a sense of contentment and fulfillment.

February 3:

Mind-

"Believe deep down in your heart that you are destined to do great things." ~Joe Paterno

Body-

Eat slowly, chew thoroughly and have a calm and relaxing atmosphere while eating. If you are angry or upset, do not eat. Drink instead. Drinking warm tea will soothe your system. Once you are calm, then you can eat your solid food.

Spirit-

Because God is faithful, we need not be afraid. God is always present and always watching over us. Say a prayer of thanksgiving.

February 4:

Mind-

Celebrate this day! Why wait for a special occasion to celebrate when you can celebrate each day. You don't need balloons, streamers

and cake to celebrate. Instead, break out in a
dance right there in your living room.

Body-

Research shows that the more multitasking you
try to do, the harder it is for you to stay focused
on any single task. Focus on the task at hand
before moving on to the next project.

Spirit-

I don't have to see visions to be aware of thy
nearness. I don't have to achieve saintliness to
know thy love.

February 5:

Mind-

The sun never sets on the fun in your family.
From birthdays to school days, it never gets dull.
And if the gray clouds creep on to the horizon,

you will keep shining, because there is always a silver lining.

Body-

There is a reason pasta has always been a go-to fuel for athletes: it's low in fat and delivers quick energy in the form of easy-to-digest carbohydrates.

Spirit-

"There comes a special moment in everyone's life, a moment for which that person was born. In that moment he finds greatness. It is his finest hour."

~Winston Churchill

February 6:

Mind-

"To effectively communicate, we must realize that we are all different in the way we perceive the world and use this understanding as a guide to our communication with others." ~Anthony Robbins

Body-

Potassium is an essential enzyme for the body's growth and maintenance tasked with managing the normal water balance between cells and body fluids Bananas are a great source of potassium.

Spirit-

Without determination you don't have any fuel for your dreams.

February 7:

Mind-

If you aren't sure of your purpose, just do what you do well, and then watch God confirm you by blessing your endeavors.

Body-

While there is no known cure to completely banish cellulite, there are ways to help minimize its appearance. By eating a healthy diet, you can help reduce cellulite. First, avoid too much sugar, which gets stored in fat cells and causes them to expand. Second, limit salt intake, since sodium causes fluid retention, making cellulite appear even worse.

Spirit-

What a blessing a drink of pure water is when one's weary steps begin to falter. Just as a runner needs to stay hydrated by drinking fluids, Christian's need to read the Bible to stay fueled.

February 8:

Mind-

Many things in life will catch your eyes, but only a few will capture your heart-pursue those.

Body-

In Native American tribes that practice smudging, herbs such as sage and lavender are burned in order to purify places of negative energy. Negative energy can be disastrous to a person's life. It can cause general bad luck, health problems, etc. Often, when a person thinks that they are cursed or hexed, the real problem is negativity.

Spirit-

"A person without a spiritual path is a person walking in darkness. With a path, we are no longer afraid or worried. "

~Thich Nhat Hanh, Buddhist monk

February 9:

Mind-

Inaction is an action, just not the kind that serves you. Sitting on the couch feeling sorry for yourself doesn't solve anything. Call a friend to meet for coffee.

Body-

Meditation-whether it involves chanting, breathing, visualization, or all the above-can be an effective stress management tool for many people. Meditation reduces stress and lowers your blood pressure.

Spirit-

In uncertain times Christ offers us certain hope. God may not solve your problems, but He will give you the strength needed to work through the issues.

February 10:

Mind-

We are on a continuum. Progress, not perfection! Use your mistakes to learn.

Body-

Brown rice is an excellent source of magnesium,
iron, and vitamin B. It is delicious with chicken
and veggies, but for optimum health benefits, try
serving it with black beans. Both brown rice and
black beans are incomplete proteins that, when
combined, provide all the nine essential amino
acids your body needs.

Spirit-

Your time is now. Embrace the now with power.
Have you been putting off a project? Now would
be a good time to tackle it.

February 11:

Mind-

I recognize my goodness and my bright inner
light. I love me.

Body-

Top turkey burgers with some capsaicin rich peppers or Tabasco sauce. Capsaicin is a spicy compound found in foods like chili peppers, jalapenos, and Tabasco sauce that is known to fight against fat and decrease inflammation.

Spirit-

See the light of Christ in every face. One Christian can spot another one in the crowd by their demeanor, speech, and actions. Make sure you are wearing a Christlike face by smiling at others.

February 12:

Mind-

"It's kind of fun to do the impossible."

~Walt Disney

Body-

To help prevent drastic spikes and drops in blood sugar, your meals and snacks should be based around lean protein, healthy fats, and unrefined carbohydrates. That means loading up on brown rice, whole grain bread and pasta, whole oats, and, of course, fruits and vegetables.

Spirit-

Regardless of what we see, God is working to fulfill Scripture's promise.

February 13:

Mind-

Gratitude is the grace of life. Make it a point to thank a family member today for something they did for you unexpectedly.

Body-

Having short- and long-term goals and races on your calendar will help you out the door. Commit yourself by signing up for a spring walk/run event.

Spirit-

The best journey you can take is the one of self-discovery. Do some soul searching today to learn more about you. On a blank piece of paper list five positive things you like about yourself. List one characteristic you would like to improve and then list the first three steps you need to take to start improving.

February 14:

Mind-

You don't get in life what you want; you get from life what you are. Work hard to make good things happen.

Body-

Don't let more than four hours go by without eating. Eating even a little something stimulates the secretion of a hormone called peptide YY-36, which reduces ghrelin production and shuts off your appetite. Also, never eat a carb with a protein. Protein slows digestion and keeps blood sugar stable. The combo helps you feel full longer, making you less likely to snack.

Spirit-

Life's worries, the deceitfulness of riches, and the lure of pleasures can combine to suffocate us spiritually.

February 15:

Mind-

If we can forget about our little aches and pains, our little personal trials, and tribulations, if we can get ourselves off our own minds and go find somebody else to help, our lives are going to get better.

Body-

Research has consistently shown that dropping just a few pounds can have a substantial impact on your blood pressure. Permanently shedding as little as five or ten pounds can decrease your risk.

Spirit-

God has placed certain people in each of our lives to help us. If we do not receive their help, we become frustrated and overworked, and they feel unfulfilled because they are not using their gifts.

February 16:

Mind-

We all have a purpose for being here. Perhaps your purpose is to be the best grandmother, or best bus driver. Figure out what your purpose is by asking, "What am I here for?"

Body-

Among adults, diabetes is the leading cause of blindness in the United Staes. Diabetes patients should go for regular eye examinations and report any changes in their vision to their doctor. Symptoms of oncoming diabetic blindness include blurry vision, sudden loss of vision, seeing dark spots in front of the eyes, having trouble focusing when reading, seeing rings around lights,

Spirit-

"The fullness of joy is to behold God in everything." ~Julian of Norwich

February 17:

Mind-

Just breathe! Excitement and anger can increase
your heart rate. Take slow, deep breaths to
lower it.

Body-

Fruits and vegetables are major sources of
potassium, so we need to work them into every
meal to get at least seven servings each day.
Make half your plate fruits and vegetables.

Spirit-

Just as a candle can help you navigate a dark
room; one spark of illumination can resolve
many of life's unanswered questions.

February 18:

Mind-

Joy and enjoyment are available just as misery is available. Choose joy. Do something for yourself today. Relax with your favorite book and a cup of tea.

Body-

Harvard studies completed over the past twenty years show the Kuna Indians drink up to forty cups of natural cocoa per week and have less than 10 percent of heart disease compared to their neighbors on the mainland. Have a piece of dark chocolate for an afternoon pick me up.

Spirit-

The family of God includes everyone for whom Jesus died. That means you!

February 19:

Mind-

In order to change and grow you need to get out of your comfort zone. Do you consider yourself lacking in technology skills? Sign up for a computer class.

Body-

Endorphins are a cluster of neurotransmitters that cause a reaction in the opiate receptors; they are the body's natural painkiller. When released, endorphins initiate a reactionary response within the body, interrupting the messages normally sent to the brain. Instead of feeling pain or stress, a feeling of euphoria is experienced.

Spirit-

"And do not forget to do good and to share with others, for with such sacrifices, God is pleased."
~Unknown

February 20:

Mind-

God is changing the world, one person at a time. Be open to change. Sometimes it adds some spice to a dull routine.

Body-

Tart cherry juice is rich in melatonin, the sleep hormone that regulates and resets your internal clock. Drink an eight-ounce glass in the morning and two hours before for sweet dreams. To get the full benefit, drink this juice at a scheduled time every day.

Spirit-

We cross each other's paths for a reason, whether as an opportunity to learn something new or heal something old. Target someone you find interesting and make sure your path crosses. It will be interesting to find out more about that person.

February 21:

Mind-

I will celebrate what is as opposed to worrying what should be.

Body-

Walnuts, flaxseeds, canola seeds, avocados, olives, and sesame seeds make some of the healthiest oils. Try this salad dressing recipe: half cup of red vinegar, one and a half teaspoons of sea salt, half a teaspoon of white or black pepper, one and a half cups of extra virgin oil (or your favorite oil listed above).

Spirit-

God looks at each of us through eyes filled with love. Be God-like today by approaching others with eyes filled with love.

February 22:

Mind-

Change your mind, and your life will follow.
Decision-making is hard because you may be
afraid of making a mistake. Once you decide, go
with it and make it work.

Body-

Dynamic stretching increases range of
movement, blood, and oxygen flow to soft
tissues prior to exertion. The dynamic exercises
you incorporate into your warmup program
should be appropriate to the movements you
would experience in your sport/event. In all the
exercises breathe easily while performing them.

Spirit-

A day's most important meetings may not be the
ones we have put on our calendar. Even though
work is done, your day is not over until you have
said good night to God through prayer.

February 23:

Mind-

"One friend in a lifetime is much; two are many; three are hardly possible."

~ Henry Brooks Adams, journalist, and novelist

Body-

Dried currants are a good source of potassium to fend off muscle cramps and keep blood pressure in check. Try substituting dried currants for raisins in your favorite cookie or muffin recipe.

Spirit-

Friendship with God is our highest calling.

February 24:

Mind-

Don't let your feelings control life. Controlling your emotions doesn't mean ignoring them. It means you recognize them and act on them when you deem appropriate, not randomly and uncontrollably.

Body-

It's never too late to quit smoking. Quitting can slow disease and increase survival odds even in smokers who have already caused significant damage to their lungs, like those with early lung cancer or COPD. Call the Tobacco Quitline at 1-800-QUIT-NOW

Spirit-

We find peace when we place our present and our future in God's hands.

February 25:

Mind-

Don't take life too seriously; no one gets out alive. Humor lightens your burdens, inspires hope, connects you to others and keeps you grounded, focused and alert.

Body-

Dietary protein is crucial in the rebuilding and recovery process, but in and of itself, protein does not build muscle. Your body builds muscle naturally in response to strenuous activity so challenge your muscles to grow by developing an exercise schedule. Decide which exercise you will do on which day. Some exercises focus on

Spirit-

Find out the needs of those near you and pray for them. Decide on one specific person to pray for today.

February 26:

Mind-

Some things in life are certain. Tomorrow's another day. Someone somewhere loves you. Going through the day with a positive attitude should be added to your list of certainties.

Body-

Boiling frozen vegetables causes vital nutrients to leach out into the cooking water. Steam, roast, or microwave them instead. Almost any hard, solid vegetable can be roasted. Good choices include peppers, squash, brussels sprouts and root vegetables.

Spirit-

God wants us to be humble and ask for help. Pride doesn't get you anywhere. God is waiting for you to ask him for help. He wants to help.

February 27:

Mind-

"Start by doing what's necessary, then what's possible, and suddenly you are doing the impossible." ~Francis of Assisi

Body-

Metabolism is vital to the long-term maintenance of a healthy weight. Some of the most important recent breakthroughs in obesity research are related specifically to metabolism. You can overcome your metabolism to lose weight and keep it off by reassessing your energy balance (you may need to eat less as you lose weight because your body needs fewer calories to sustain itself).

Spirit-

God is the answer. The question doesn't matter.

February 28:

Mind-

Work like you don't need the money.

Love like nobody has ever hurt you.

Dance like nobody is watching.

Sing like nobody is listening.

Live as if this was paradise on earth.

Body-

Foods that are red, yellow, orange, green, and purple are low in calories and are loaded with vitamins and minerals your body needs to function, keep your immune system up, and maintain strong bones and muscles.

Spirit-

Everything in our lives can be used to serve God. What special talent do you have? Use it today to serve God.

February 29:

Mind-

I am a tower of power, rebuilding my body and taking charge of my life. I have accomplished sixty days of change; I only have 305 to go.

Body-

Physical activity remains important for all who want to lose weight, as it helps you to burn the calories that you consume each day. Creating a calorie deficit remains the easiest way to lose weight and exercising daily will help you to create this deficit. Exercise can include a walk around the block.

Spirit-

Live gently and responsibly in gratitude for the world God has given us. It took God six days to create the world, what better way to say thank you than by volunteering in a community service project today.

March 1:

Mind-

March is Optimism Month. Do one nice thing to make someone else smile every day this month. Bet it will make you feel pretty good too!

Body-

When we are sleep deprived, we may feel the need to eat more, which can lead to weight gain. The answer is to get eight hours of sleep.

Spirit-

Jesus is the bread of life. The bread of life is the spiritual food you need in order to live spiritually. Just as physically you need to eat in order to live, the bread of life gives you nourishment for the soul.

March 2:

Mind-

I am not fully dressed until I adorn myself with a smile. Keep up your positive attitude. Winter is almost over, and spring will be here soon.

Body-

Metabolism boosting vitamin B also helps prevent heart disease and cancer. There are nine B vitamins that all assist in losing weight. Vitamin B can be found in nuts, legumes, fruits, and vegetables. If you control total calories, eating a handful of nuts is a great snack. Besides holding you over until dinnertime you will be gaining health benefits.

Spirit-

Generosity is a way of life that goes beyond money. God gave us many talents. Figure out which talent you can share with someone else.

March 3:

Mind-

There are only some things you encounter in life that can be changed. Focus on the things that can be changed.

Body-

Eat lightly cooked vegetables because you digest them more slowly. Both fruits and vegetables contain soluble fiber. As a rule, vegetables make better sugar blockers, because they have more fiber and less sugar. Roasted vegetables like cauliflower can often serve as a delicious starch substitute.

Spirit-

It's too easy to get caught up in life's dramas and forget about the big picture, but when you reach out and help someone, you feel your sense of purpose and mission kick in.

March 4:

Mind-

You can't finish the race until you take the first step. Because spring is so close you are probably excited about spending time outside. Find a community walk to benefit your favorite charity scheduled for early summer

Body-

Wild berries have superb antioxidant capacity and have demonstrated a remarkable ability to lower blood glucose levels for diabetics.

Spirit-

Today, look for God's presence in every situation. Even when you are upset with a situation, look to God for guidance in solving the issue peacefully and gracefully.

March 5:

Mind-

Find a way to serve someone who usually serves you.

Body-

Chili peppers contain capsaicin, a compound that gives spicy peppers their zing. Capsaicin also curbs your appetite while you eat and raises your body temperature, which may boost your metabolism. Find a way to add chili peppers to one of your meals today. They add zest and color as well as health benefits.

Spirit-

When we listen, we will hear God speak. We may not hear what we want to hear but he will speak.

March 6:

Mind-

Little acts of kindness can add up to a lifetime of happiness. Commit a random act of kindness today by doing something nice for someone.

Body-

As many as 283 species of bacteria can thrive in ordinary office dust, including streptococcus, the main cause of strep throat. Wipe down your workstation, keyboard, and phone regularly with a disinfectant.

Spirit-

Great spiritual teachers do not always wear robes and live in temples or lecture halls. Strive to be a teacher today by acting Christlike.

March 7:

Mind-

Laugh, laugh often, laugh when you want to cry, and laugh at yourself.

Body-

Dried blueberries are rich in falconoid, a class of antioxidants that may boost brain functioning. Make a batch of blueberry oatmeal cookies substituting dried blueberries for the raisins.

Spirit-

Thank God for every ordinary day.

March 8:

Mind-

Now is the time to renew your commitment to unlocking the potential of girls and women everywhere. Celebrate women today, International Women's Day.

Body-

A one ounce serving of avocados gives you a natural, creamy texture with nearly twenty vitamins and minerals and only fifty calories per serving. An easy way to get a one-ounce serving is to add sliced avocado to a lettuce salad.

Spirit-

When we follow Jesus faithfully, our words and actions will match.

March 9:

Mind-

"If I had a flower for every time you made me smile and laugh, I'd have a garden to walk in forever." ~Author Unknown

Body-

For a grain to be considered whole, it must contain all three nutrient-packed parts of the grain seed: the outside shell or bran, the inside or endosperm, and the heart or germ. The refining process removes the bran and germ along with naturally occurring fiber, iron, and B vitamins.

Spirit-

"Let your light shine before others, so that they may see your good works and give glory to your Father in heaven." ~Matthew 5:16

March 10:

Mind-

"Love is not what the mind thinks, but what the heart feels." ~Greg Evans

Body-

Tart cherry juice, which relieves soreness, is often blended with sweet fruits. For the most cherry antioxidants, choose brands without other fruit and buy 100 percent fruit juice so there's no added sweetness. Remember, when there is added sweetness that equals added calories.

Spirit-

No matter how long it takes us to turn toward home, we can trust that God will welcome us there.

March 11:

Mind-

Our greatest glory is not in never falling but in rising every time we fall.

Body-

If you work at home, it's just you and fridge-and nobody watching. Because you have no meetings or structured activities, you can check the mail, toss in a load of laundry, play with the dog, and grab a snack (or two or four). To prevent this, keep a log of your daily activities, including every time you get up to eat. If you still feel the need to snack, eat at the kitchen table-and don't do anything else.

Spirit-

Listen to the voice of God, who seeks our good and cheers us on.

March 12:

Mind-

A smile is contagious. When you smile at someone else it improves your mood as well as the other person.

Body-

A cup pf valerian tea with honey before bed is a centuries-old practice. The natural compounds in valerian tea have been used as a sedative and may help reduce the amount of time it takes you to fall asleep. The glucose in honey will help you relax as you are trying to fall asleep; it affects orexin, a neurotransmitter that has been linked to alertness.

Spirit-

"When Jesus spoke again to the people, he said, "I am the light of the world. Whoever follows me will never walk in darkness but will have the light of life." ~John 8:12

March 13:

Mind-

Friends are the most important ingredient in the recipe of life.

Body-

While you don't want to overdo it, eating an egg or two a few times a week isn't dangerous. In fact, eggs are an excellent source of protein and contain unsaturated fat, a so-called good fat. Poached eggs are perfect because they are easy to make and have no added fat.

Spirit-

When we walk in the light of Christ, we grow into who God wants us to be.

March 14:

Mind-

Dream! It is important to have a dream, something to work towards. Make a list of your forgotten dreams. Perhaps one of them is achievable at this point in your life.

Body-

When you eat is an important as what you eat for a peaceful night. Eating late at night forces your body and brain to digest instead of resting. Avoid eating three hours before going to bed.

Spirit-

Sing with all your heart. Remember, God doesn't care if you are tone deaf. He just wants to hear you sing.

March 15:

Mind-

If you want to leave a mark, you must *make* a mark. Do something big that is noticeable and beneficial to others.

Body-

If you have trouble applying eye shadow or concealer because of yellowish eyelid bumps, the problem may be more than just cosmetic. People with eyelid bumps also have higher levels of bad LDL cholesterol and triglycerides, and lower levels of good HDL cholesterol. Make sure your doctor peeks at your face while your eyes are closed.

Spirit-

Let us consider how to provoke one another to love and good deeds.

March 16:

Mind-

You cannot grow and expand your capabilities to their limits while running the risk of failure.

Body-

Family friendly snacks should include low-calorie foods that are high in water or fiber and aren't loaded with fat. Go with fruits such as grapes or berries or fix some air-popped popcorn.

Spirit-

Live in such a way that those who know you but don't know God will come to know God because they know you.

March 17:

Mind-

Happiness comes from within and is found in the present moment by making peace with the past to looking forward to the future!

Body-

A single potato provides a hefty dose of potassium and 35 percent of your daily vitamin C needs. Enjoy a baked potato with your lean protein. Instead of smothering it with sour cream and butter, try a spoonful of salsa. You will be adding flavor with the calories from fat.

Spirit-

"Jesus said, 'Have I not commanded you? Be strong and courageous. Do not be terrified; do not be discouraged, for the Lord your God will be with you wherever you go." ~Joshua 1:9

March 18:

Mind-

I don't suffer from insanity; I enjoy every minute of it. Life is sometimes chaotic so just go with the flow.

Body-

Avoid cottonseed and soybean oil when buying mayonnaise, margarine, and dressings. They are high in omega-six fatty acids, which cause inflammation. Daily consumption of these fatty acids is common because they are hidden in oils and processed food.

Spirit-

Faithful disciples are proof that Christ lives.

March 19:

Mind-

Every ending can open onto a new beginning.

Body-

Whole grains are intact kernels loaded with health-promoting bran, fiber, vitamins, and minerals (particularly the B vitamins, vitamin E, magnesium, and zinc), and various antioxidants. The general rule of thumb is to pick carbohydrates where the first ingredient on the label has the word "whole" in it-100 percent whole wheat, whole oats, etc.

Spirit-

Every little thing is going to be all right. Sometimes God uses pain to inspect us, correct us, direct us, and perfect us.

March 20:

Mind-

Know your heritage. Know it beyond all reason and beyond all doubt. No one can take that from you. Spend time researching your family tree.

Body-

More and more studies are reporting tangible health benefits for coffee drinkers. Drinking coffee regularly can help protect your heart and liver, reduce your risk of dementia, Alzheimer's, Parkinson's disease, and diabetes, and may even relieve your headache. Avoid adding cream and sugar thus avoiding calories.

Spirit-

God splashes through life's puddles close beside me. He is never far from your side, so in times of crisis or stress, reach out for him and he will offer support.

March 21:

Mind-

No matter how long the winter, spring is sure to follow. It is always easier to have a positive attitude when the grass is green, and the songbirds are singing. Congratulations, you survived winter.

Body-

Research shows that people with apple-shaped bodies (with more weight around the waist) face more health risks than those with pear-shaped bodies who carry more weight around the hips. Belly fat has been linked to an increased risk of heart disease and diabetes.

Spirit-

If we acknowledge God's constant presence in our lives, God always leads us on the right path.

March 22:

Mind-

How you frame something can change everything. Try to consider the sunny side of a situation rather than focusing on the negative.

Body-

Energy levels will decrease if carbohydrate intake is limited or carbohydrate stores in the body are low. You need energy to fuel your activities. A piece of fresh fruit is perfect for a morning or afternoon snack.

Spirit-

"I've often thought, 'I'm nobody.' But God's not impressed by eloquence; he's impressed by out longing for him." ~Stormie Omartian, author

March 23:

Mind-

"Be an optimist. There is not much use being anything else." ~Winston Churchill

Body-

Vitamin D is a critical vitamin when it comes to fighting off colds. It also promotes absorption of calcium for bone health, boosts immune function, and reduces inflammation. An eight-ounce glass of low fat or skim milk is a great source of vitamin D.

Spirit-

If we pay attention, moments in every day will call us to worship.

March 24:

Mind-

To grow, you need to step outside your comfort zone. Write a letter to the editor of the newspaper expressing your opinion on a local matter.

Body-

A recent study found that tomato paste and olive oil boosts pro-collagen, a molecule that gives the skin its structure and keeps it firm and youthful. An Italian dish of pasta would be perfect for dinner to reap the benefits of younger looking skin.

Spirit-

"Therefore, my heart is glad, and my glory rejoiceth: my flesh also shall rest in hope."
~Psalm 16:9

March 25:

Mind-

"I think I would rather possess eyes that know no sight, ears that know no sound, hands that know no touch than a heart that knows no love." ~Author Unknown

To feel loved by another person is the ultimate natural high. Be sure to let a special person in your life know you love them.

Body-

Scientists say that mundane tasks, such as entering data into a spreadsheet, can switch your mind into default mode, making you more likely to mess up within thirty seconds. Feel like you are operating on autopilot? Snap out of it by going for a quick walk down the hall.

Spirit-

God is at work to mend the brokenness with us.

March 26:

Mind-

"You can't have everything. Where would you put it?" ~Steven Wright, stand-up comedian, and actor

Body-

Potassium is an essential mineral your body needs to regulate your blood pressure. Studies suggest that getting ample amounts of potassium can help keep blood pressure under control, as well as fend off stroke and heart disease. Figs are a great source of potassium. However, be aware that too much potassium is toxic, so get what you need from food, not supplements.

Spirit-

Jesus died for all people.

March 27:

Mind-

"At birth our divine potential is folded up in us like a tent. It is life's purpose to unfold that tent." ~Hildegard of Bingen

Body-

Researchers found that eating with one other person increased the size of each diner's meal by 28 percent. Two extra diners increased everyone's meal size by 41 percent, and six or more dinner partners led each to consume 76 percent more food. Eating with a group may cause people to linger and eat more than they would if they were alone. Eating alone all the time can be lonely so eat with others occasionally but be aware of what and how much you eat.

Spirit-

God accepts me and declares me beloved.

March 28:

Mind-

It's never too late or too early to start something new. Why wait to start a resolution on the first of January when every day is appropriate for a new start?

Body-

If you have knee pain, raising your seat by a few inches can make a difference. You won't have to bend your knees as much to sit down, which will make it a lot easier to get back up.

Spirit-

With God a "no" can be a step toward something even better.

March 29:

Mind-

"What lies behind us and what lies before us are tiny matters compared to what lies with us." ~Ralph Waldo Emerson

Body-

Getting enough protein daily is essential for your overall health. Healthy protein sources include eggs, nuts, lean meats, fish, dairy, and certain grains.

Spirit-

"Is any one of you sick? He should call the elders of the church to pray over him and anoint him with oil in the name pf the Lord." ~James 5:14

March 30:

Mind-

Play with abandon. Have you ever watched a child play? They have so much energy and do not care if anyone sees them being silly. Play like a child today and have fun.

Body-

Oolong tea boosts metabolism, helping you burn fat faster. Studies have shown that drinking oolong teas has led to sustained weight loss and a smaller waist size. Be careful not to drown your tea in sugar, which will negate the benefits.

Spirit-

Live with intention.

March 31:

Mind-

A genuine smile communicates compassionate caring, true kindness, and a humble attitude.

Body-

Eat at least seven servings of fruit and vegetables daily. Emphasize the vegetables, especially leafy greens like romaine lettuce, spinach, swiss chard, collards, and fresh sprouts.

Spirit-

God never, ever gives up on us.

April 1:

Mind-

Live healthy; live happy. Have a family member join you on a walk today.

Body-

Running hills develops efficiency, endurance, and power. Ascending an incline uses more muscle fibers than running on level terrain, and climbing longer hills makes the body recruit muscles when they're fatigued, which helps develop your finishing speed.

Spirit-

"This is the confidence we have in approaching God: that if we ask anything according to his will, he hears us." ~1 John 5:14

April 2:

Mind-

Without confidence we are stifled at every turn.

Body-

Americans have the highest cholesterol in the world. Too much cholesterol in your bloodstream can have several serious effects on your overall health, such as contributing to hardening of your arteries or narrowing of the arteries, which can cause constrictions to the flow of blood. This in turn can have serious implications for your general health and for your heart health and can lead ultimately to your death from heart attack. A healthy diet and exercise can lower your cholesterol.

Spirit-

Be the light of Christ to all you meet.

April 3:

Mind-

"Remember, the greatest gift is not found in a store, nor under a tree, but in the heart of true friends." ~Cindy Lew

Body-

Static stretching is a form of stretching that involves moving to a held position and holding this position for about fifteen to thirty seconds, followed by a slow release of the held position. Static stretching is recommended only after resistance training or physical activity. An example is lying on your back with one leg held extended at right angles to the body.

Spirit-

We do not need to be perfect to be used by God!

April 4:

Mind-

Always strive for success. Study what works, evaluate why it works and replicate the effort to get the same excellent results in everything you do.

Body-

Sleep helps us thrive by contributing to a healthy immune system and can also balance our appetites by helping to regulate levels of the hormones ghrelin and leptin, which play a role in our feelings of hunger and fullness.

Spirit-

"But store up for yourselves treasures in heaven, where moth and rust do not destroy, and where thieves do not break in and steal. For where your treasure is, there your heart will be also."
~Matthew 6:20-21

April 5:

Mind-

If you want a life of purpose and meaning, you must *live* with purpose.

Body-

For a creamy indulgence, Greek style yogurt contains the same number of calories as regular fat-free yogurt (one hundred per cup) but twice the protein and half the carbs. Its velvety texture makes a great base for dips, too.

Spirit-

We need to do the best we can to hear from God, then decide based on what He has said to us.

April 6:

Mind-

"The most completely lost of all days is the one in which we have not laughed." ~French proverb

Body-

Complex carbs like whole grain pasta offer a steady supply of tryptophan, an amino acid used to make the mood-lifting brain chemical serotonin. Tryptophan is one of the ten essential amino acids that the body uses to synthesize the protein it needs. Tryptophan helps regulate your appetite, helps you sleep better and elevates your mood.

Spirit-

When we commit our ways to God, God commits heaven's resources to us.

April 7:

Mind-

When life's music starts playing, you're ready to dance. There's a celebration in each new day, and your eyes are open to catch it. It all puts a smile on your face, and you're ready to share.

Body-

Donating blood has obvious benefits to the recipients, but there are also lesser-known benefits to the donor. IF you donate blood on a regular basis, you can get more than just a great feeling that you saved a life. You are also helping to save your own. You get the benefit of becoming very aware of your body, facts like your blood type, cholesterol, blood pressure and iron levels.

Spirit-

God's love will sustain us through all our tomorrows.

April 8:

Mind-

Dance in the rain.

Body-

Think outside the sports-drink bottle when you are looking for a workout beverage. New research puts the spotlight on beet juice. Exercise feels easier due to the nitrates. Nitrate in the beet juice is converted by bacteria living on the tongue into the chemical nitrite. Once it enters the stomach, it becomes nitric oxide or re-enters the blood stream as nitrite. The nitrites work by protecting against endothelial dysfunction, which means that blood vessels have trouble expanding or contracting to handle changes in blood flow.

Spirit-

It is our responsibility to share with those who are not as richly blessed.

April 9:

Mind-

"Love is not blind. It sees more and not less, but because it sees more, it is willing to see less."
~Will Moss

Body-

Five ways to lower your cholesterol:

1. Trim belly fat by eating five to six small meals to boost your metabolism.
2. Exercise every day.
3. Eat five to seven fruits and vegetables daily.
4. Eat one cup of oatmeal daily.
5. Take one teaspoon of psyllium daily (Metamucil).

Spirit-

"He makes me lie down in green pastures, he leads me beside quiet waters, he restores my soul. He guides me in paths of righteousness for his name's sake." ~Psalm 23:2-3

April 10:

Mind-

Catch up with a friend from years past. Call someone you haven't spoken to in a year or two. Just calling to say hi will feel good to both of you.

Body-

Diets high in refined sugar can cause indigestion and trigger insulin surges that interfere with the hormones that affect sleep. The solution: low-fat and high-fiber foods such as fruit and vegetables.

Spirit-

God never gives up on anyone.

April 11:

Mind-

Spend time with people you respect and who embody the qualities you want to have and learn from them.

Body-

You can reap more cardio benefits by picking up the pace within some of your runs. Do eight to ten surges lasting fifteen to thirty seconds.

Spirit-

"This is what the Lord says: 'Stand at the crossroads and look; ask for the ancient paths, ask where the good way is, and walk in it, and you will find rest for your souls.'" ~Jeremiah 6:16

April 12:

Mind-

What fills the heart shows in the face.

Body-

Traditional Indian sauces can be high in sodium, so look for those with less than three hundred milligrams per serving. Tasty Bite Tikka Masala Simmer Sauce is shipped directly from India and has been applauded for low sodium content.

Spirit-

We are all children of the earth.

April 13:

Mind-

Every action, no matter how small, can cause a huge reaction somewhere else or at some future time.

Body-

Eating healthy is an important component to living a long and disease-free life. But any healthy diet also allows for some indulgence. When you deprive yourself of your favorite food, your diet will fail. Use self-control rather than deprivation.

Spirit-

"it's simple: when you haven't forgiven those who have hurt you, you turn your back against your future. When you do forgive, you start walking forward." ~Tyler Perry, actor, producer, and director

April 14:

Mind-

One way to foster a positive attitude is to cultivate an attitude of gratitude.

Body-

If you do something for thirty days, it becomes a habit. If you do something for forty days, it becomes a routine. If you do something for ninety days, it becomes a lifestyle.

Spirit-

"Peace I leave with you, my peace I give unto you: not as the world giveth, give I unto you. Let not your heart be troubled, neither let it be afraid. ~John 14:27

April 15:

Mind-

To forget how to dig the earth and tend the soil
is to forget ourselves.

Body-

To hit your salt craving, try popcorn. Baked
tortilla chips have 110 calories in a once ounce
bag. One ounce of air-popped popcorn (no
butter) has the same number of calories but
more volume, yielding four cups and five grams
of fiber.

Spirit-

Through Christ's wounds we are healed.

April 16:

Mind-

Performing at your highest level requires risk taking and pushing yourself outside your comfort level. If you have been walking around the block on a regular basis, try walking two blocks. If you have been running a mile on a regular basis, try running two miles.

Body-

Running has an uncanny ability to mellow the soul, take the edge off hard feelings, and put things back into healthy perspective. Running is a great stress reliever and may even relieve mild depression.

Spirit-

"But those who hope in the Lord will renew their strength. They will soar on wings like eagles; they will run and not grow weary; they will walk and not be faint." ~Isaiah 40:31

April 17:

Mind-

Asking for guidance and heeding it is a mark of wisdom.

Body-

With the right ration of run/walk segments, almost anyone can finish a marathon (26.2 miles) without pain. To run or walk a marathon, the technique doesn't mean walking when you get tired; it means taking brief walk breaks when you're not.

Spirit-

"Thus you will walk in the ways of good men and keep to the paths of the righteous. For the upright will live in the land, and the blameless will remain in it." ~Proverbs 2:20-21

April 18:

Mind-

Go deep! Yes, go deep...reach deep within yourself to tap into all your strengths. Go deep with your goal, don't just look at the surface of its impact, and look for its long-term and lasting effect.

Body-

Frankincense, an aromatic resin used in incense and perfumes is used to treat lung and Genito-urinary complaints, ulcers, chronic diarrhea, breast cysts, and excessive menstruation. It can also be used for acne and fungal infections. Frankincense essential oil is obtained by steam distillation of the dry resin and is used in aromatherapy.

Spirit-

Even if reconciliation is not possible, God can help us to forgive.

April 19:

Mind-

"When one door of happiness closes, another opens; but often we look so long at the closed door that we do not see the one which has opened for us." ~Helen Keller

Body-

Women whose diets are rich in olive oil have less skin damage and wrinkles. If you lack oil in your diet, experience the benefits through olive oil skin care products. Olive oil skin care was discovered over five thousand years ago and quickly became an essential component of skin care. The benefits are obvious when we observe the beautiful skin of Mediterranean women.

Spirit-

"Teach us to number our days aright that we may gain a heart of wisdom." ~Psalm 90:12

April 20:

Mind-

"The value of love will always be stronger than the value of hate." ~Franklin D. Roosevelt

Body-

To make your sandwich succulent, instead of mayo, try spreading your next sandwich with a few thin slices of avocado. You will still get the rich flavor and creamy texture, but with fewer calories and the benefit of good fats.

Spirit-

"Pray continually." ~1 Thessalonians 5:17

April 21:

Mind-

"Life begins outside your comfort zone."
~Unknown

Body-

One of the hardest parts of losing weight is giving up your favorite foods-so why not give them a healthy makeover instead? Swap in more nutritious ingredients to lower sodium, fat, and sugar. The result? Healthy, delicious meals that will satisfy you and power your workouts without derailing your weight loss efforts.

Spirit-

"And as for you, brothers, never tire of doing what is right." ~2 Thessalonians 3:13

April 22:

Mind-

Good works flow from a grateful heart.

Body-

Wild salmon provides a substantial dose of mega-three fatty acids, also known as the good fats, which contains alpha-linolenic acid, an organic compound that helps keep skin smooth and supple by building connective tissues and strong cell membranes. A popular way to prepare wild salmon is to grill it. Flavor salmon with your favorite seasonings, cover with aluminum foil. Do not overcook the salmon.

When it changes color and can be flaked with a fork your fish is done. (Check after ten minutes of grilling.)

Spirit-

A lot of kneeling will keep you in good standing.

April 23:

Mind-

Happiness is a state of mind.

Body-

"Do you not know that in a race of the runners run, but only one gets the prize? Run in such a way as to get the prize. Everyone who competes in the games goes into strict training. They did it to get a crown that will last forever." ~1 Corinthians 9:24-25

Spirit-

We never outlive Christ's call to serve others.

April 24:

Mind-

Practicing regular meditation is one of the best ways to bring stress hormone levels back to normal quickly. One type of meditation is guided meditation. With this method you form mental images of places or situations you find relaxing. You try to use as many senses as possible, such as smells, sights, sound, and textures.

Body-

Aroma therapists use Eucalyptus to aid respiratory system ailments by enhancing deep breathing. It is recommended for muscle aches and pains.

Spirit-

When you pray, think beyond the hospital visitation list.

April 25:

Mind-

Don't spend your life trying to do what you are not gifted to do. Focus on a talent you possess and share it with someone. Perhaps you knit or crochet and can teach someone else.

Body-

The tea from the prickly Nettle plant helps to prevent hay fever and allergy attacks by blocking the histamines in your body. Nettle tea is dense, so brew it for fifteen to twenty minutes. Make a larger pot during allergy season and keep it in the fridge. Add lime to freshen the taste.

Spirit-

Whether or not we get to see it, every act of love bears fruit.

April 26:

Mind-

"If you could achieve any one goal in your life within twenty-four hours, which goal would have the greatest impact on your life?" ~Brian Tracy

Body-

Recovery days make your training count because your body makes fitness gains while you're at rest. Time is one of the best ways to recover from a workout. Your body has an amazing capacity to take care of itself if you allow it for some time. Resting and waiting after a hard workout allows the repair and recovery process to happen at a natural pace.

Spirit-

God can lead us from death and destruction to life and hope.

April 27:

Mind-

"Your work is to discover your world and then with all your heart give yourself to it." ~Budda

Body-

Chronic stress releases cytokines and C-reactive protein in your body-dangerous molecules that cause inflammation and put you at greater risk for developing arthritis, irritable bowel syndrome, and other chronic diseases. Try a massage as a stress reliever. Regular massage may reduce blood pressure in people with hypertension and may lead to less pain, depression, and anxiety.

God has surprises in store for us every day.

April 28:

Mind-

"Winning does not always mean coming in first...Real victory is in arriving at the finish line with no regrets because you know you've gone all out." ~Apolo Anton Ohno, Olympic champion speed skater

Body-

Each tender stalk of roasted asparagus is a source of folic acid, a natural mood lightener. Dip the spears in fat free yogurt or sour cream for a hit of calcium with each bite.

Spirit-

Neither a job nor a bank account is the source of our security; God is.

April 29:

Mind-

"It is amazing what you can accomplish if you do not care who gets the credit." ~Harry S. Truman

Body-

Used in traditional Chinese medicine (TCM) as a tonic, the herb *Schisandra* helps to restore a weak immune system, increase mental focus, and improve physical stamina. Schisandra can be found in capsule form wherever vitamins and supplements are sold.

Spirit-

"Faith goes beyond reason. It goes beyond what you can see. But it is as real as anything you can touch or feel." ~Henry Cloud, author

April 30:

Mind-

Laughter is like a medication; it keeps us lighthearted; it also keeps us connected with others.

Body-

About 90 percent of all diabetics represent type two diabetes. Research indicates that nearly 75 percent of all new cases of type two diabetes could have been prevented through doing regular exercise or physical activity while maintaining normal weight values. Are you keeping up with your exercise, so you do not become a statistic?

Spirit-

"In the happy moment, praise God. In the difficult moments, seek God. In the quiet moments, trust God. In every moment, thank God." ~Robert Albert Wood

May 1:

Mind-

"Tact is getting your point across without stabbing someone with it." ~Shirley Zieve

Body-

Short on time? Use intervals to get stronger more quickly. To increase your endurance, four to six thirty-second bursts of all-out cardio is just as effective as up to an hour of training at a lower intensity. This is also a good variance to your routine in order to avoid boredom.

Spirit-

"Jesus said, 'I tell you the truth, anyone who gives you a cup of water in my name because you belong to Christ will certainly not lose his reward." ~Mark 9:41

May 2:

Mind-

"A vacation is having nothing to do, and all day to do it in." ~Robert Orben, magician, and writer

Body-

Tart cherry juice is the ultimate antioxidant because it relieves pain, fights heart disease, and works as a sleep aid. Enjoy an eight-ounce serving today.

Spirit-

We can be set free from our past when we place our future in God's hands.

May 3:

Mind-

"Some of the greater things in life are unseen; that's why you close your eyes when you kiss, cry, or dream." ~Author unknown

Body-

1. Yogic breathing exercises reduces blood pressure in people with hypertension, possibly through their effects on the automatic nervous system, which governs heart rate, digestion, and other largely unconscious functions.

2. Empty your lungs by breathing out through your nose.
3. Inhale slowly through your nose while you silently count to five.
4. Exhale slowly and steadily through your nose. Tensing your stomach muscles can draw out the last of your breath.
5. Continue the pattern of slow, focused inhaling and exhaling for ten cycles.

Spirit-

"When life knocks you on your knees, you're in the perfect position to pray!" ~Anonymous

May 4:

Mind-

While words may fail us, the Holy Spirit never does. You may only be someone in the world, but to someone else, you may be the world.

Body-

Allergy symptoms peak in the early morning, when adrenaline and cortisol levels are low, allowing inflammation to occur. The action of a twenty-four-hour antihistamine peaks at twelve hours, so taking it in the evening should blunt the worst symptoms the next morning. However, decongestants are better taken in the morning because they can disrupt your sleep.

Spirit-

Jesus made sure He had seasons of peace and alone time. He ministered to the people, but He slipped away regularly to be alone and pray. Seek some quiet time for yourself today.

May 5:

Mind-

"If people concentrated on the really important things in life, there would be a shortage of fishing poles." ~Doug Larson, American columnist

Body-

Want to lose weight for good? The key is exercising consistently in a way that burns calories, reduces body fat, builds muscle, and stokes your metabolism. With spring comes nice weather inviting us outside. A good way to stay active is through gardening and yard work. Mow your lawn using a push mower, prepare your garden for planting. Stay busy!

Spirit-

God leads us into the future one step at a time.

May 6:

Mind-

Every time a smile breaks across your face, the entire energy of your body lifts.

Body-

Cutting too many carbs, calories, or grams of fat to lose weight could shortchange you of crucial vitamins and minerals. For maximum energy, more than half your daily calorie intake should come from carbohydrates, preferably complex ones such as whole grain cereal and whole-wheat pasta. Your daily intake will depend on how strenuous your exercise regime is.

Spirit-

When we know we are obeying God, we can endure whatever comes at us.

May 7:

Mind-

"The most desired gift of love is not diamonds or roses or chocolates. It is focused attention."
~Rick Warren, founder of Saddleback Church, Lake Forest, CA

Body-

Ask your doctor to run a cholesterol test twice a year, once in the summer and then again in

December when cholesterol peaks. Average the two readings to get the best picture of your cholesterol levels year-round.

Spirit-

"Jesus replied, 'What is impossible with men is possible with God.'" ~Luke 18:27

May 8:

Mind-

"Children may close their ears to advice but may open their eyes to example." ~Patricia Hoolihan, author

Body-

Exhaustion is not simply lack of sleep; it is related to stress, dehydration, nutrition, and lifestyle. Conquering your exhaustion can feel insurmountable, but it could be as simple as listening to music, having more sex, or changing the way you breathe.

Spirit-

Stop struggling; our Lifeguard is always on duty. God always takes care of us.

May 9:

Mind-

Love is louder than the pressure to be perfect. Unconditional love is a term that means to love someone regardless of one's actions or beliefs. It is a concept comparable to true love.

Body-

The key to lunch isn't just what you eat, but when you eat. You should eat your midday meal

at the same time every single day. Working through the lunch hour, only to wolf down something at three in the afternoon sends your hormones into a tizzy. It throws your body's natural circadian cycle out of whack for the rest of the day.

Spirit-

"Faith is not believing God can; it is knowing that he will." ~Ruth Park

May 10:

Mind-

Happy people live longer. Find what makes you happy. After all, you are responsible for your own state of happiness.

Body-

Eat a variety of fruits and vegetables to obtain the widest selection of nutrients that boost immunity, beautify skin, accelerate fat loss, increase energy, prevent heart disease, and fight cancer. Fill half of your plate with vegetables such as carrots, broccoli, and salad.

Spirit-

"Jesus said to them all, 'If anyone would come after me, he must deny himself and take up his cross daily and follow me.'" ~Luke 9:23

May 11:

Mind-

"No matter what accomplishments you achieve, somebody helped you." ~Althea Gibson, Wimbledon tennis championship

Body-

Antioxidants are higher in black raspberries than other berries. Select plump, well-colored blackberries. They should not have stem caps

attached. If hulls are still attached, the berries
are immature and picked too early. Avoid berries
showing any signs of decay. When buying
berries, shop with your nose. Always pick the
plumpest and most fragrant berries. They should
be firm, bright, and fresh looking with no mold
or bruises.

Spirit-

True discipleship asks us to walk a difficult road.

May 12:

Mind-

You can't change the past, but you can always
look toward the future. Accepting and even
anticipating change makes it easier to adapt and
view new challenges with less anxiety.

Body-

Deep breathing can help you...
1. Clear your mind.
2. Reduce stress and anxiety.

3.   Be more in the present moment.
Take a minute and add this practice into your daily routine. 4-7-8 Breathing Technique:
1.   For a count of 4 seconds.
2.   Hold for a count of 7 seconds.
3.   Exhale for a count of 8 seconds.
4.   Repeat these steps 3x in a row.

Spirit-

There is no need for temples, no need for complicated philosophies. My brain and my heart are my temples; my philosophy is kindness. ~Dalai Lama

May 13:

Mind-

"What lies behind us and what lies before us are tiny matters compared to what lies within us." ~Ralph Waldo Emerson

The kind of person you are on the inside is what is important. Strive to be loving and kind.

Body-

Even a ten-to fifteen-minute run will improve your vitality and boost your mood due to the release of endorphins.

Spirit-

"I believe in Christianity as I believe that the sun has risen. Not only because I see it, but because I see everything by it." ~C.S. Lewis

May 14:

Mind-

Don't stress over things you can't control. Your performance is based on your training, not on external things.

Body-

Deep breathing is important for relaxed eating. Also important is the speed in which you eat.

Some tips for creating a relaxed environment at mealtime include:

1. Dine with eating companions who nourish and inspire you.
2. Light a candle at the table, play quiet music, make your table inviting by using centerpieces and placemats.
3. Notice your posture as you eat. A straight spine allows for fuller, deeper breaths.

Spirit-

"Each person is born with a calling. It is your task to discover what that calling is and find a way to make that calling a reality." ~Lucy MacDonald

May 15:

Mind-

"Be more concerned with your character than with your reputation, because your character is what you really are, while your reputation is merely what others think you are." ~John Wooden

Body-

Though sage is most used in cooking, sage tea has been shown to boost alertness and mood while decreasing anxiety. It also has flavonoids that reduce inflammation. To enhance the flavor, mix it with black tea, brew it for five to ten minutes, and add a pinch of honey.

Spirit-

"Keep on loving each other as brother. Do not forget to entertain strangers, for by so doing some people have entertained angels with knowing it." ~Hebrews 13:1-2

May 16:

Mind-

"We look forward to the time when the Power of Love will replace the Love of Power. Then will our world know the blessings of peace." ~William Ewart Gladstone

Body-

Avoid common breakfast mistakes such as skipping breakfast to lose weight, not eating enough protein, skimping on fiber, taking in too many or too few calories, not reading food labels and drinking too many calories. Your breakfast should consist of 1 serving of protein,1 serving of grain, and a serving of fruit or vegetable.

Spirit-

Spiritual sayings for contemplation and meditation are a good way to focus on the positive when you begin to feel bombarded with negativity. Start your list today.

May 17:

Mind-

There comes a time when you must stand alone. You must feel confident enough within yourself to follow your own dreams. You must be willing to make sacrifices.

Body-

A cup of steamed asparagus contains just fifty calories and provides 115 percent of your daily value for vitamin K-a nutrient that is critical for healthy bones and tissue.

Spirit-

We cannot do anything or everything that everyone else is doing. But we can do everything God has called us to do.

May 18:

Mind-

True gifts come with no strings attached.

Body-

Easy runs let your muscles recover while improving your biomechanical efficiency, which translates into improved running form.

Spirit-

"The measure of a Christian is not in the height of his grasp but in the depth of his love." ~Clarence Jordan

May 19:

Mind-

"It's no trick loving somebody at their best. Love is loving them at their worst." ~Tom Stoppard, playwright

Body-

Find a group of fun friends to train with, that way you can share advice, push each other in workouts, and enjoy the journey together and make some great memories along the way!

Spirit-

"There is a time for everything, and a season for every activity under heaven: a time to be born and a time to die, a time to plant and a time to uproot." ~Ecclesiastes 3:1-2

May 20:

Mind-

"What you are thunders so that I cannot hear what you say to the contrary." ~Emerson

Body-

You can improve your run if you cross-train once a week to strengthen connective tissue and areas like the Achilles tendon. Cross training refers to an athlete training in a sport other than the one that athlete competes in with a goal of improving overall performance. For example, if you are a marathon runner, try bike riding as a cross training sport.

Spirit-

"Faith is not merely hope, and it must be more than belief, faith is a knowing of the heart."
~Rev. Floyd and M. Elaine Flake, authors

May 21:

Mind-

Happy people have higher energy. It is thought that happy people have stronger romantic and social relationships than others and it all stems from a philosophical view of life.

Body-

This week see whether you can incorporate a regular relaxation period into the midafternoon of every day. Even fifteen minutes will be a good benefit. Try to close off the outside world, close your eyes, breathe, and recharge.

Spirit-

"Live a balanced life-learn some and think some and draw and paint and sing and dance and play and work every day some." ~Robert Fulghum

May 22:

Mind-

Regardless of how distant your dreams may seem, every second counts.

Body-

Staying hydrated is one of the easiest things you can do for energy. Proper hydration is important for overall health. Insufficient hydration fatigues your muscles, reduces your coordination, and causes muscle cramps.

Spirit-

"If your happiness depends solely on external possessions and circumstances, your boat, in the sea of life, will inevitably turn to the safety of the harbor over and over again, and you will miss the joy of sailing towards the unknown." ~Lucy MacDonald

May 23:

Mind-

The only time a lazy man ever succeeds is when he tries to do nothing.

Body-

Just two strength-training sessions per week can improve your running. Strength training is the use of resistance to muscular contraction to build strength, endurance, and muscles. There are many different methods of strength training. Lifting weights is a form of strength training. Lifting weights is a form of strength training. For beginners, you want to choose about 8-10 exercises, which comes out to about one exercise per muscle group.

Spirit-

God can use our failures to bring new growth.

May 24:

Mind-

We often get hung up on things like not having enough money or education, living in the wrong city, not having the "right" clothes, a lack of technology...the list of perceived disadvantages is limited only by your imagination.

Body-

After hard or long runs (two hours or more), eat carbs and protein within thirty minutes to restock energy stores and rebuild muscles. Try a whole-wheat bagel or a handful of dried figs.

Spirit-

"The key to release, rest, and inner freedom is not the elimination of all external difficulties. It is letting go of our pattern of reactions to those difficulties." ~Hugh Prather

May 25:

Mind-

Inspiration comes from within.

Body-

A diet rich in vitamin C and linoleum acid, a fatty acid found in many vegetable oils, can reduce the appearance of wrinkles, dryness, and thinning skin. As we age, our skin loses moisture and elasticity, making it prone to wrinkles. Take measures to protect your skin against wrinkles by protecting your skin from the sun and wearing sunglasses regularly.

Spirit-

"Dream as if you'll live forever; live as if you will die today." ~James Dean

May 26:

Mind-

Don't spend your life hating someone who is probably out having a good time while you are upset.

Body-

To keep the intensity low on your easy days, avoid running with fast friends. Head out by yourself, or schedule a fun, social run with a slower runner. Remember a slow run is at a comfortable pace.

Spirit-

"To forgive is the highest, most beautiful form of love. In return, you will receive untold peace and happiness." ~Robert Muller

May 27:

Mind-

Confidence is generally described as a state of being certain either that a hypothesis or prediction is correct or that a chosen source of action is the best or most effective. Self-confidence is having confidence in yourself.

Body-

Digestive and calorie burning metabolism are strongest when the sun is highest in the sky (lunchtime) and weakest in the late evening. This is why European countries make the noon meal the biggest meal of the day.

Spirit-

Each time you face a choice today, pause for a few seconds to consider how your decision can serve God's purpose.

May 28:

Mind-

It isn't the man who takes things as they come
that succeeds but the man who also grabs them
as they go.

Body-

Currently as much as 70 percent of the American
population is estimated to simply disregard the
advice related to physical activity and are at risk
to become part of the estimated 435,000
premature deaths each year, arising from a
sedentary lifestyle or poor diet.

Spirit-

"Faith is not simply a patience that passively
suffers until the storm is past. Rather, it is a spirit
that bears things with blazing serene hope."
~Corazon Aquino, former president of the
Philippines

May 29:

Mind-

If you aim to make every workout perfect, you end up spending valuable time and energy recovering from the inevitable disappointment.

Body-

Women need other women to feel creative, to laugh with and explore life with. Creating a bond with other women creates a rich space in our lives. Who are your friends and what are you doing to foster that all-important friendship?

Spirit-

"Brothers, I do not consider myself yet to have taken hold of it. But one thing I do: Forgetting what is behind and straining toward what is ahead, I press on toward the goal to win the prize for which God has called me heavenward in Christ Jesus." ~Philippians 3:13-14

May 30:

Mind-

"A friend is a person with whom I may be sincere. Before him I may think aloud." ~Ralph Waldo Emerson

Body-

If practice races wear you out, scale back expectations for your big event. Start conservatively and pick up the pace near the end only if you're feeling great.

Spirit-

God's love covers all our sins.

May 31:

Mind-

What doesn't kill you will only make you stronger.

Body-

In January millions of Americans resolve to lose weight, and by Memorial Day 8- percent have failed. It is not too late to recommit for the summer.

Spirit-

"Show me your ways, O Lord, teach me your paths."

June 1:

Mind-

"Time spent laughing is time spent with the gods." ~Japanese Proverb

Body-

Research shows drinking moderate amounts of red or white wine with a meal can help lower your risk of developing heart disease and diabetes.

Spirit-

Christ breaks the shell around our heart to set us free and heal us.

June 2:

Mind-

"Let us endeavor to live, so that when we die, even the undertaker will be sorry." ~Mark Twain

Body-

Single genes and clusters of genes probably make some people more likely to develop diabetes when they gain weight, while others can add pounds and not develop diabetes. The longer you live with diabetes, the more likely you are to develop complications. If you develop diabetes at a young age, the chances are greater of complications at a younger age. Diabetes will shorten your life. To prevent, or lessen your chances of being diagnosed with diabetes, lose weight, exercise, and eat healthy.

Spirit-

We find our purpose in life by serving and loving those around us.

June 3:

Mind-

"I don't know anyone who enjoys failure or setbacks. But it's precisely those times when we get stronger and learn the most about ourselves." ~Edward Grinnan, author

Body-

Kiwi fruit contains about seventy milligrams of vitamin C-more than an orange and just five milligrams short of the daily recommendation for women. The flavor of a kiwi can be described as a cross between strawberries, bananas, and pineapple and can be eaten raw or cooked.

Spirit-

"Faith isn't the ability to believe what you can see. It's the ability to see what you believe." ~LeRoy A. Chappelle

June 4:

Mind-

"Love is never quite as satisfying as when we give it away." ~Doris Ann Dillon

Body-

When running uphill, keep your head and chest up, drive with your arms, and run with high knees. On downhills, your feet should land underneath you, not in front, so shorten your stride slightly.

Spirit-

"People are like stained glass windows. They sparkle and shine when the sun is out, but when the darkness sets in, their true beauty is revealed only if there is a light from within." ~Elisabeth Kubler-Ross

June 5:

Mind-

"Greatness is making others feel great!" ~G.K. Chesterton

Body-

Sometimes the company of a friend can be one of the strongest motivators to exercise. Invite a friend to workout with you. If there is someone else depending on you, you will be less likely to back out of the workout.

Spirit-

Through Christ peace is possible.

June 6:

Mind-

The simple act of smiling activates happiness centers in the brain.

Body-

There's a good reason we crave chocolate when we are sad and depressed. Tryptophan boosts mind-lifting serotonin in the brain. A study found that even the taste, texture, and smell make us happy.

Spirit-

Jesus died for you and you and you-and me.

June 7:

Mind-

"Let us be grateful to people who make us happy; they are the charming gardeners who make our souls blossom." ~M. Proust

Body-

Clothing manufacturers adjust their measurements, so women feel better and spend more. The trend is toward bigger sizes being labeled with smaller and smaller numbers as clothing designers add inches to the traditional sizes. The trend is called "vanity sizing" and occurs when a size twelve dress might be labeled an eight. Manufacturers can pick whatever measurement they want and attach a number to it.

Spirit-

Claiming Jesus as Lord is only the beginning of faith.

June 8:

Mind-

"Don't let success go to your head-and if you fail, don't let failure go there either." ~Jane Seabrook and Ashleigh Brilliant, authors

Body-

It's okay to multitask when it comes to finding time to squeeze in a workout. Find something you like to do while you catch up on your favorite TV series. You can work out on an exercise ball or lift dumbbells, ride a stationary bike, or walk. The opportunity for movement is endless so be creative.

Spirit-

"Jesus said to Martha, 'I am the resurrection and the life. He who believes in me will live, even though he dies; and whoever lives and believes in me will never die. Do you believe this?" ~John 11:25-26

June 9:

Mind-

"Challenges are but achievements yet to be accomplished." ~Norm Duesterhoeft, captain, retired United States Army

Body-

Upper-body exercises help swimmers develop the strength and endurance necessary to push and pull through water's resistance lap after lap. There is a large range of upper body workouts that you can do at home. It is always smart to warm up your muscles before working them and then try the following: triceps dips, push-ups, triceps pushup and pull-ups.

Spirit-

"If anyone is in Christ, he is a new creation; the old has gone, the new has come!" ~2 Corinthians 5:17

June 10:

Mind-

"Wherever you go, no matter what the weather, always bring your own sunshine." ~Anthony J. D'Angelo

Body-

Healthy eating will give you confidence in your nutrition and help you feel like an athlete. It is all about the positive attitude you have adopted. If you feel good about yourself, you are going to communicate that to others. It all starts with a balanced diet.

Spirit-

Spiritual hunger and spiritual thirst, like physical hunger and thirst, are common to all.

June 11:

Mind-

"When it comes time to go after a goal, starting the belief system early will create the mental road map the body can follow leading up to the event." ~Terrence Mahon, Olympic coach

Body-

Rosemary can be used to soothe sore muscles as well as improve your memory. Use the herb to make a body scrub to relieve aching muscles and smell it to boost your brain power.

Spirit-

"Life is either a daring adventure or nothing. To keep our faces toward change and behave like free spirits in the presence of fate is strength undefeatable." ~Helen Keller

June 12:

Mind-

Life is short-break rules, forgive quickly, kiss slowly, love truly, laugh uncontrollably, and never regret anything that made you smile.

Body-

To speed up recovery, have a glass of low fat or fat free chocolate milk after running longer than forty-five minutes. The protein found in chocolate milk helps repair damaged muscle and build new, lean muscle.

Spirit-

"Take the first step in faith. You don't have to see the whole staircase, just take the first step."

~Dr. Martin Luther King Jr.

June 13:

Mind-

Create something special. Being creative alters us by improving our mood, self-esteem, and socialization. Creativity can take many forms. It is not black or white, simple, or complex; it is an approach and an attitude of coloring your world differently.

Body-

Swimming exercises almost the entire body-heart, lungs, and muscles-with very little joint strain. It is great for general fitness, just not a great way to drop excess pounds.

Spirit-

Each day is an opportunity to live the adventure of giving.

June 14:

Mind-

I breathe easy knowing I am surrounded by positive energy, healing feelings, and people who love me.

Body-

We are all metabolically different. The only way to determine your unique needs is to experiment. If you don't have time for a more substantial relaxed lunch, it might be useful to have a smaller lunch and then a substantial late-afternoon snack. Think of it as two lunch meals.

Spirit-

God wants you to give your will to Him. Just give Him your will, your mind, your heart, your all.

June 15:

Mind-

May you have enough happiness to make you sweet, enough trials to make you strong, enough sorrow to keep you human, and enough hope to make you happy.

Body-

Eating quality food is perhaps the most powerful and foolproof nutritional strategy you can choose. Higher quality food means greater nutritional value. When you continually eat low quality food, the brain will register a nutrient deficit and signal you to eat more.

Spirit-

"If it is contributing to the needs of others, let him give generously; if it is leadership, let him govern diligently; if it is showing mercy, let him do it cheerfully." ~Romans 12:7-8

June 16:

Mind-

It's not what you see, but how you choose to see it that counts. Look for the good in yourself. Look for the good in others. Look for the good in your situation. Look for the good in life.

Body-

Tai chi (a Chinese martial art) combined with qigong (Chinese yoga) is more than just a gentle way to work out. Practicing these ancient disciplines can reduce stress and have a powerful effect on metabolic syndrome. These arts can reduce systolic and diastolic blood pressure and trim your waist size by at least an inch. Tai chi is sometimes described as "Meditation in motion" and can burn as many calories as moderate intensity activities such as walking.

Spirit-

In every dark place, look for light from God.

June 17:

Mind-

"Every day there is an opportunity to excel. Unfortunately, most folks just stand there idle." ~Norm Duesterhoeft, captain, retired United States Army

Body-

Because of the type of deep breathing that's incorporated into yoga, when you do even a single pose, you bring oxygenated blood to your organs. The goal of yoga, or of the person practicing yoga, is the attainment of a state of perfect spiritual insight, and tranquility while meditating.

Spirit-

God invites us to draw near, just as we are.

June 18:

Mind-

"It is a happy talent to know how to play."

 ~Ralph Waldo Emerson

Body-

"The higher your energy level, the more efficient your body. The more efficient your body, the better you will feel and the more you will use your talent to produce outstanding results."
~Anthony Robbins

Spirit-

"When you come to the end of the light you know, and it's time to step into the darkness of the unknown, faith is knowing that one of two things shall happen; either you will be given something solid to stand on, or you will be taught to fly." ~Edward Teller

June 19:

Mind-

"The beauty of compassion is that every one of us already possesses it. We are born with our arms reaching out to embrace." ~Tim Sanders, author

Body-

For your best chance of a successful race, aim for more than one worthy goal. Many runners will plot out new race times or distances to work towards. Others will chip away at their fifty-state dream or travel to an exotic race location. All of these are worthy goals and are the things that keep us moving forward.

Spirit-

"The foundation of good is always love."

~J. Philip Wogaman, former president of Interfaith Alliance

June 20:

Mind-

Friends are flowers in the garden of life.

Body-

The type of fiber in potatoes keeps your intestinal tract muscles working and blocks a small amount of caloric absorption. In fact, research shows that men and women who eat fiber from vegetables like potatoes have less body fat and smaller waist. The fiber content of a potato with skin is equivalent to that of many whole grain breads, pastas, and cereals.

Spirit-

"Love must be sincere. Hate what is evil; cling to what is good. Be devoted to one another in brotherly love. Honor one another above yourselves." ~Romans 12:9-10

June 21:

Mind-

"Love and kindness are never wasted. They always make a difference. They bless the one who receives them, and they bless you, the giver." ~Barbara De Angelis, PhD, author of self-help books

Body-

Scientists can't decide whether being overweight is a disease, a symptom, a risk factor for other diseases, a nonissue that will have no ill effect on health, or perhaps even a slightly positive indicator for longevity. The answer is that carrying extra weight is all of these.

Spirit-

"Awake, north wind and come, south wind! Blow on my garden that its fragrance may spread abroad." ~Song of Song 4:16

June 22:

Mind-

If you think you will be happy once you lose ten pounds, be happy now. If you imagine you will have more energy when you finally eat right, have more energy now.

Body-

Developing a training plan can improve the quality of your workout and enhance your performance. Sticking to a training plan is good- if you are healthy. Cut back on mileage or take a rest day if you feel extra tired or sore. Stay flexible; let your body dictate what it is ready for.

Spirit-

"When you believe that you cannot stitch your own heart back together, go to work on the hearts of other people; there is no surer way to repair yourself than to repair them." ~Andrew Solomon

June 23:

Mind-

Act as if you are the person you wish to be and you will not only convince the rest of us, but you will also prove it to yourself.

Body-

Pomegranates help reduce inflammation that causes soreness and weakness. It is the seed of the fruit that you want to use in your recipes.

Spirit-

"The best thing to give to your enemy is forgiveness; to an opponent, tolerance; to a friend, your heart; to your child, a good example; to a father, deference, to your mother, conduct that will make her proud of you; to yourself, respect; to all men, charity." ~Benjamin Franklin

June 24:

Mind-

Friendships must be intended and tended.

Body-

Make solo runs pleasant by picking scenic routes and a sunny day. Even varying something so simple as the route offers a change of pace to prevent boredom.

Spirit-

"Even if he lives a thousand years twice over but fails to enjoy his prosperity. Do not all go to the same place?" ~Ecclesiastes 6:6

June 25:

Mind-

I need to devote myself to making things turn out fine.

Body-

People actively engaged in leisure or occupational physical activity, as well as those who participate in activities that are physical in nature for the specific goal of improving fitness, are at a lower risk for mortality from sudden cardiovascular disease. This sounds like reason enough to add activity to your day. Who wouldn't want to live longer?

Spirit-

"Affirm continuously to yourself; I am in the right place, at the right time, for the right purpose." ~Ursula Roberts

June 26:

Mind-

By changing the way you portray your circumstances to yourself and others, you change their emotional effect.

Body-

A single dose of exercise works even better than tranquilizers as a muscle relaxant among individuals with symptoms of anxiety and tension. But without any undesirable effects.

Spirit-

Choosing God's way is an ongoing process.

June 27:

Mind-

"Slow down and enjoy life. It's not the scenery you miss by going too fast-you also miss the sense of where you are going and why." ~Eddie Cantor

Body-

Mediterranean cuisine is not only one of the most flavorful diets in the world, but thanks to a wealth of delicious fresh ingredients, it is also one of the healthiest. It is vegetable dominant with the most prevalent ingredients being olive oil, eggplant, artichokes, squash, and tomatoes with grilled meat used sparingly.

Spirit-

"Not everyone who says to me, 'Lord, Lord,' shall enter the kingdom of heaven, but he who does the will of my Father who is in heaven." ~Matthew 7:21

June 28:

Mind-

You can discover more about a person in an hour of play than in a year of conversation." ~Plato

Body-

Fruit smoothies are a versatile way to add fruits and other healthy foods to your diet. Some tips for making delicious yogurt smoothies include:

1. Blend the fruit long enough but not too long. Blending too long will remove nutrients and flavor.
2. Use honey instead of sugar. Honey has a higher sweetener power than sugar and provides vitamins and minerals.
3. When possible, use plain natural yogurt. This will enhance the flavors you add.

Spirit-

"For God so loved the world that he gave his one and only Son, that whoever believes in him shall not perish but have eternal life." ~John 3:16

June 29:

Mind-

Believe and achieve! If you have made up your mind that you can't do it, you are right.

Body-

You can lose up to one to two liters of sweat per hour of exercise in warm weather. Hydrate pre-run with sixteen ounces of a sports drink, which will provide quick energy. Most sports drinks contain electrolytes, carbohydrates, potassium, and vitamins. Your body will absorb the fluid from sports drinks at a faster rate than water to help replenish what was lost during a workout.

Spirit-

"I have great faith that there's a master plan and that even if we don't understand it and even if it's heartbreaking, there's a reason for everything. And I hold on to that." ~Terri Irwin, widow of Steve Irwin, the crocodile hunter

June 30:

Mind-

"There is a way of perceiving that leads to cynicism and divisiveness, a closing off of possibility; and there is a way that leads to higher faith and love." ~Cynthia Bourgeault, author

Body-

One cup of green beans boasts four grams of fiber plus a healthy dose (30 percent daily value) of skin helping vitamin C. Fresh green beans straight from the garden are the best but if you are unable to obtain them, you can still get many valuable nutrients from green beans that have been frozen or canned.

Spirit-

"Faith is building on what you know is here so that you can reach what you know is there." ~Cullen Hightower, author

July 1:

Mind-

"Life is too important to be taken seriously."
~Oscar Wilde

Body-

People who run more than thirty-five miles a week are 54 percent less likely to suffer age-related vision loss than those who cover ten miles a week. Further research is needed to explore why there is a link between exercise and the decreased risk for eye disease. Findings may show that the person who runs is healthier overall.

Spirit-

"The simple act of reflecting, the simple act of pausing to consider, to reason, can have an impact." ~Dalai Lama

July 2:

Mind-

A calm mind creates a calm body. Calmness must involve the human being's whole life; inwardly and outwardly; what is apparent and what is hidden. Inner calmness is made up of tranquility of the mind, serenity of the heart and calmness of thought.

Body-

Dehydration results in premature fatigue and increases the risk of heat illness. Dehydration disturbs the body's fluid and electrolyte balance, increases stress on the heart, and contributes to the effects of excess body heat.

Spirit-

True faith lets God be God.

July 3:

Mind-

"Success is not the key to happiness. Happiness is the key to success." ~Herman Cain, newspaper columnist

Body-

Cinnamon slows the passage of food through your stomach. It also lowers your blood sugar levels by stimulating glucose metabolism. Cinnamon is a very tasty herb that has many uses. From cookies to cakes to pies you can find many uses for cinnamon. The herb, cinnamon is actually bark that is ground to a powder form or sold in a stick form.

Spirit-

"Filled with compassion, Jesus reached out his hand and touched the man. 'I am willing,' he said. 'Be clean!' Immediately the leprosy left him and he was cured." ~Mark 1:41-42

July 4:

Mind-

We need to cultivate the spirit of gratitude in our relationships, remembering to say thank you.

Body-

Research has linked diets abundant in tomatoes to lower cancer rates. Lycopene is a vital antioxidant that helps fight against cancerous cell formation. Free radicals in the body can be flushed out with it and derive its rich redness from the nutrient. It takes as littles as 540 millimeters of liquid tomato product to get the full benefits of Lycopene. This means that a daily glass of tomato juice has the potential to keep a person healthy for life.

Spirit-

"The real voyage of discovery consists not in seeking new landscapes, but in having new eyes." ~Marcel Proust

July 5:

Mind-

Feeling sure about yourself and your abilities is not only beneficial to feeling good but also has a profound impact on the social, professional, romantic, and physical aspects of your life.

Body-

Fresh basil has a sweet, pungent flavor and loads of nutrients. Two tablespoons of the chopped herb provide more than a quarter of your daily value for vitamins, A, and C, as well as calcium and iron.

Spirit-

We can trust in God's presence and provision every day.

July 6:

Mind-

"When you fail you gain experience, and with enough experience, you don't fail as often."
~Colin Powell, former secretary of state

Body-

Avoiding too much sun can head off skin cancer, and it can also keep you looking young by preventing wrinkles, fine lines, and saggy skin. Sun protection is the most important skin care product you can use every day. Sunscreen should be an SPF 15 or higher. It can be in your foundation or moisturizer, and it will help prevent new wrinkles from developing and existing ones from getting deeper.

Spirit-

At the end of life's journey, we will be greeted
by our loving Savior.

July 7:

Mind-

"Love has nothing to do with what you're
expecting to get-only with what you are
expecting to give-which is everything."
~Katharine Hepburn, actress

Body-

Raspberries are a great source of fiber-some of it
soluble in the form of pectin, which helps to
lower cholesterol. One cup of raspberries has
eight grams of fiber. Raspberries are also an
excellent source of vitamin C. Make a batch of
pancakes topped with fresh raspberries for a
refreshing start to your day.

Spirit-

"Is prayer your steering wheel or your spare tire?" ~Corrie Ten Boom

July 8:

Mind-

"If you are able to laugh, you are the owner of the world." ~Roberto Benigni, Italian comedian

Body-

When you run on an empty stomach, your metabolism gets turned on early; it keeps going longer, thus burning off more fat. Also, if you run on an empty stomach, your body is forced to use the energy that is most available to it at the time, which on an empty stomach is your body's store of fat. Make running your first activity of the day if you want to amp up those weight-loss benefits.

Spirit-

We may think our words are so tiny and insignificant that they do not matter. They may seem insignificant, but they are important.

July 9:

Mind-

"Deep faith is paranoia turned inside out...It allows us to trust ourselves and others even if we and they have proven untrustworthy in the past." ~Thomas Moore, author

Body-

If you have a jam-packed day of meetings, you can still squeeze in some exercise if you are creative. Three ten-minute segments of moderate-intensity exercise throughout the day is acceptable because it keeps your metabolism elevated. A simple way to meet this goal is to use the stairs rather than the elevator.

Spirit-

The joy, peace, and fulfillment we seek come from being filled with God, and nothing else.

July 10:

Mind-

"There is only one real failure in life, and that is not to be true to the best one knows." ~John Farrar, Australian composer

Body-

Research has proven that proper hydration before, during, and after a workout is important because it increases energy, helps regulate body temperature, assists in delivering sugar glucose to the muscles, and helps remove toxins and waste from your body. Pick up a bottle of Powerade Zero. It is a zero-calorie sports drink that helps replenish sodium, potassium, calcium, and magnesium.

Spirit-

"Our Lord did not ask us to give up the things of earth, but to exchange them for better things."
~Fulton J. Sheen

July 11:

Mind-

Intend to succeed! Success is only a matter of luck-ask any man who has failed.

Body-

Sugar snap peas are a cross between snow peas and English peas. Eaten whole, they provide two grams of fiber and just twenty-six calories in one cup. The sweet, crunchy vegetable contains 63 percent of your daily value of vitamin C, along with a good dose of iron and vitamin K, a nutrient important for bone health.

Spirit-

"You might as well try to hear without ears or breathe without lungs, as to try to live a Christian life with the spirit of God in your heart." ~D.L. Moody

July 12:

Mind-

There are five ways to smile:

1. Wake up.
2. Be thankful.
3. Be approachable.
4. Complain less.
5. Smile more.

Body-

Gardening tasks, such as weeding, raking, digging, and pruning burn 230 or more calories an hour, about the same as brisk walking. Be sure to use sunscreen of SPF 15 or higher while working outside.

Spirit-

"You will know the truth and the truth will set you free." ~John 8:32

July 13:

Mind-

Love is the only game two can play and both can win." ~Elizabeth A Kutsche

Body-

Increasing the number of steps you take per minute helps you become a more efficient, faster runner. You can practice this skill throughout the day, every day. Before you know it, you will be a faster runner.

Spirit-

"Let us not become weary in doing good, for at the proper time we will reap a harvest if we do not give up." ~Galatians 6:9

July 14:

Mind-

Endurance never sleeps. Endurance is the ability or strength to continue through fatigue and stress so there is no opportunity to slack off. You need to keep moving forward.

Body-

Spending time in nature helps restore your energy. Fresh air also helps improve your heart rate, blood pressure, and metabolism, helps your immune system fight off disease more effectively, soothes your nerves, stimulates your appetite, and will help your food to digest more effectively and it will help you sleep more soundly at night.

Spirit-

"God loves us for, and sometimes in spite of, who we are." ~William Tully, Rector, St. Bartholomew's Church

July 15:

Mind-

When you feel you need to start pointing out flaws in the world around you, perhaps you should start with a mirror.

Body-

Strengthening your trapezius muscle, which runs from your shoulders to your neck and upper back, can reduce chronic neck pain. The trapezius muscle responds well to massage. Try this self-massage on your trapezius muscle:

1. Cross one arm in front of your body so that you can place the palm of your hand on top of the other shoulder.
2. Beginning at the base of the neck, knead the muscles in a rhythmic action, moving out toward the arm in increments.
3. Relax and enjoy!

Spirit-

"Christ is a substitute for everything, but nothing is a substitute for Christ." ~Dr. H.A. Ironside

July 16:

Mind-

"A life without love in it is like a heap of ashes upon a deserted hearth, with the fire dead, the laughter stilled, and the light extinguished. ~Frank Tebbets

Body-

A pattern of consistently good sleep will give you a boost of growth hormones, which are great for rebuilding muscle fibers. Strive for seven to eight hours of sleep a night.

Spirit-

"The sun glints through the pines, and the heart is pierced in a moment of beauty and strange pain, like a memory of paradise. After that day, we become seekers. ~Peter Matthiessen

July 17:

Mind-

When we make another life better, we make our own life better. The more you extend yourself in service, the more you will cease feeling alone and insignificant.

Body-

Paddling a kayak is great exercise. Remember that it takes more energy to paddle through

water less than three feet deep because
resistance is greater in shallow water. Kayaking
is a sport that can be enjoyed by all ages but
there are some safety measures that should be
learned before venturing out on the water.

Spirit-

"If God gave you roses and then you ask, 'Why
are there no thorns?' God would just smile and
show His bleeding hands, saying, 'I took them
away to save you from pain.'" ~Anonymous

July 18:

Mind-

If you want to be successful, you must either
have a chance, or take one.

Body-

Bicycle riding enhances your quality of life both
physically and financially, but it also improves
the environment by reducing your carbon

footprint. Most car trips are single-occupancy ga-guzzlers, with a lone driver using tremendous amounts of energy to get from here to there. Bikes are perfect transportation for one person, and especially handy as a green way to cover short distances.

Spirit-

"Going to church doesn't make you a Christian any more than going to the garage makes you a car." ~Laurence J. Peter

July 19:

Mind-

"The most powerful force in business isn't greed, fear, or competition. The most powerful force in business is love." ~Tim Sanders, former chief solutions officer at Yahoo!

Body-

Swimming is a healthy activity that can continue for a lifetime. It works practically all of the muscles in the body if you perform a variety of strokes. Swimming can develop a swimmer's general strength, cardiovascular fitness, and endurance. Breaststroke, backstroke, butterfly, and crawl are the most popular swim strokes.

Spirit-

When we are like Jesus, we show God to the world.

July 20:

Mind-

"If you ask me what still keeps me here on this earth, what keeps me alive then I would answer without hesitation; love." ~Imre Kertesz, Auschwitz survivor

Body-

Your ideal running week will include a longer run to build endurance, a hilly run to improve your strength, and scenic or social run that regularly injects fun into your routine and keeps you coming back for more.

Spirit-

"No matter how good we are, God could love us no more. And no matter how bad we are, he could love us no less." ~Mike Huckabee, former Arkansas governor

July 21:

Mind-

Live. Love. Laugh. Acquire enthusiasm; you can't be enthusiastic and unhappy at the same time.

Body-

When you want to engage in good self-control, the best thing that you can do for yourself is set

up your day, so you exert your self-control resources toward that specific task you want to succeed at. For example, if you decide to cut back on the amount of candy you eat you do not want a dish of candy staring you in the face first thing in the morning. Move it out of eyesight.

Spirit-

"How else but through a broken heart may Lord Christ enter in?" ~Oscar Wilde

July 22:

Mind-

Happiness is not a destination in which you arrive. It is your journey there. Whatever benefits you expect to be yours at the end of your journey, simply receive them in the beginning.

Body-

Diets high in refined sugar can cause indigestion and trigger insulin surges that interfere with the hormones that affect sleep.

Spirit-

"A person does not have to be behind bars to be a prisoner. People can be prisoners of their own concepts and ideas. They can be slaves to their own selves. ~Maharaji

July 23:

Mind-

The best and most beautiful things in the world cannot be seen or even touched. They must be felt with the heart.

Body-

Some studies suggest that DHA levels in the brain decrease with advancing age and that humans with senile dementia treated for six months with fish-oil capsules (1400 milligrams of DHA per day) show improvement in intellectual function.

Spirit-

"Live as though Christ died yesterday, rose from the grave today, and is coming back tomorrow."
~Theodore Epp

July 24:

Mind-

Hanging on to resentment is letting someone you despise live rent-free in your head.

Body-

No matter what your experience with bicycling is, riding a bike can be a great way to get healthy exercise. Even small increases in activity will produce measurable health benefits. You can ride a bicycle almost anywhere, at any time of the year, and without spending a fortune. Most of us know how to bike and once you have learned you don't forget. All you need is a bike, a helmet, and a half hour here or there and a bit of confidence.

Spirit-

When we commit ourselves to prayer, we open ourselves to a changed life.

July 25:

Mind-

Live with purpose. A man with enterprise accomplishes more than others because he goes ahead and does it because he is ready.

Body-

Even moderate exercise-a quick thirty-minute walk each day, for example-can lower your risk of heart problems. Other easy ways to incorporate exercise into your day is to park at the end of the parking lot and walk from there instead of driving around looking for the closet spot. You can also use the stairs instead of the elevator. Always be conscious of opportunities to move.

Spirit-

Your spirit needs nourishment just like your body does. Don't wait until you have a crisis in your life to start feeding it.

July 26:

Mind-

I feel in harmony with the universe and secure with myself.

Body-

Red-, yellow-, and green-colored sweet peppers add a painter's palette of colors to meals, along with a healthy dose of vitamins A and C. Roasting or grilling intensifies their flavor and gives them a creamy texture.

Spirit-

Even though we are not perfect, we can be strong.

July 27:

Mind-

Tell yourself that you can achieve your goals and say it out loud if that helps. It may sound corny, but if you think you can't do something, you probably won't.

Body-

Studies show that insomniacs fell asleep in seventeen minutes on days they ran, compared to thirty-eight minutes on days they didn't. They also slept for an extra hour on days they exercised.

Spirit-

"Sometimes your medicine bottle has on it, "Shake well before using." That is what God has to do with some of His people. He has to shake them well before they are ever usable." ~Vance Havner

July 28:

Mind-

A good mantra diverts your mind from thoughts that reinforce the pain to thoughts that help you transcend it.

Body-

A vegetarian diet is not by definition a healthy one. You can't just replace meat with French fries. What makes a great vegetarian diet is eating whole foods that come from the earth like whole grains, fruits, vegetables, beans, and nuts. Beans are the ultimate source of protein, and they are loaded with fiber.

Spirit-

God is good even when our lives don't seem to be.

July 29:

Mind-

"All of us are responsible for one another."
~Talmud

Body-

Heat stroke is a form of hyperthermia in which the body temperature is elevated dramatically. Heat stroke is a medical emergency and can be fatal if not promptly and properly treated. Cooling the victim is a critical step in the treatment of heat stroke. The most important measure to prevent heat stroke is to avoid becoming dehydrated and avoid vigorous physical activities in hot and humid weather.

Spirit-

God can speak through our acts of kindness.

July 30:

Mind-

When we demonstrate love or compassion or concern, we are walking in the footsteps of

spiritual giants; we are fulfilling our highest
potential as human beings.

Body-

Aroma therapists use lavender essential oil to
treat rheumatism, sprains, respiratory problems,
abdominal cramps, depression, insomnia,
tension-related problems, burns, and various
types of skin infections. Lavender flowers can be
candied and are sometimes used as cake
decorations. Lavender flavors baked goods and
desserts and is also used to make lavender
sugar.

Spirit-

"Faith is like electricity. You can't see it, but you
can see the light." ~Gregory Dickow, pastor

July 31:

Mind-

"Be faithful in small things, because it is in them that your strength lies." ~Mother Teresa

Body-

For a nutritional boost, add to your smoothies a few teaspoons of flaxseed oil, which is rich in inflammation-reducing omega-three fatty acids. Try this strawberry banana smoothie for a refreshing pick me up: one and a half cups plain yogurt, two bananas (cut up), half a cup fresh or frozen strawberries, two tablespoons of wheat germ, one tablespoon of honey and two teaspoons of flaxseed oil. Combine the ingredients in a blender and blend until smooth.

Spirit-

Even though we are not perfect, we can be strong.

August 1:

Mind-

When you give, you strengthen a mind-set of abundance rather than one of lack. Service makes you feel good. It helps you transcend the small self in favor of the higher Self.

Body-

Don't forget to drink at least eight glasses of pure water every day. When you don't get enough water, the result is added stress on all of the organs and cells in the body.

Spirit-

Give the Lord your will, your love, your life, your self, your all, and find the joy and peace that passes all understanding.

August 2:

Mind-

"You never climb higher than the ladder you select." ~Italian proverb

Body-

Regular swimming builds endurance, muscle strength, and cardiovascular fitness. It can serve as a cross training element to your regular workouts. Using swimming as a cross training activity allows the runner to have a break from running without taking a day completely off from exercise.

Spirit-

Prayer opens the door for God's power and strength to fill us.

August 3:

Mind-

"If you're lucky enough to have done well, then it's your responsibility to send the elevator back down." ~Kevin Spacey, actor

Body-

Blueberries are often called a "superfood." This small but mighty berry is loaded with nutrients. They may help lower blood pressure, prevent heart disease, improve memory, aid in exercise recovery, and more.

Spirit-

In the hour of severe trial, happy is that person whose God is the Lord.

August 4:

Mind-

"Success without honor is an unseasoned dish; it will satisfy hunger, but it won't taste good." ~Joe Paterno, Penn State football coach

Body-

It is estimated that one in five Americans will be affected by some form of skin cancer during his or her lifetime, and exposure to ultraviolet (UV) rays is the most preventable risk factor. Easy steps like applying sunscreen, wearing sun-protective clothing, and seeking shade all help to lessen your skin cancer risk.

Spirit-

Anything that connects us to God is a form of prayer.

August 5:

Mind-

"Successful people are those who've fallen off the horse a dozen times and gotten back on a dozen times." ~Jean Driscoll, wheelchair racer

Body-

When you are stressed, your body produces a surge of hormones, like adrenaline and cortical, which may cause a temporary spike in blood pressure by making your heartbeat faster and your blood vessels narrow.

Spirit-

"It is not how much we do, but how much love we put in the doing. It is not how much we give, but how much love we put into the giving." ~Mother Teresa

August 6:

Mind-

"Decisions and discipline can't be separated; one is worthless without the other." ~John C. Maxwell, author, and motivational speaker

Body-

Smokers are at a higher risk of hypertension. But even though tobacco and nicotine in cigarettes can cause temporary spikes in blood pressure, smoking itself is not thought to cause chronic hypertension. Instead, factors associated with smoking, like heavy alcohol consumption and lack of exercise, might be responsible.

Spirit-

"This is my simple religion. There is no need for temples, no need for complicated philosophy. Our own brain, our own heart is our temple; the philosophy is kindness." ~Dalai Lama

August 7:

Mind-

"I don't know the key to success, but the key to failure is trying to please everybody." ~Bill Cosby, actor, and comedian

Body-

Consider walking around while talking on the phone, organizing your closet, cleaning out the garage bit by bit, setting an alarm on your computer to signal break time, or simply visiting the office water cooler more often. All are examples of how you can increase the steps you take.

Spirit-

"David wasn't thinking of being king when he was tending sheep; he was just doing what God sat before him." ~John Fisher

August 8:

Mind-

Never give up! The mighty oak was once a little nut that held its ground.

Body-

Brush walnut oil onto grilled vegetables for a slightly nutty flavor or toss a few teaspoons of it into pasta or salad. Walnut oil is an expensive, delicate specialty oil that can replace olive oil in dressing or sauce recipes, but it is not a cooking oil. It is used mainly for its rich nutty taste.

Spirit-

"Difficulties are meant to rouse, not discourage. The human spirit is to grow strong by conflict."
~William Ellery Channing

August 9:

Mind-

"A teacher ultimately is judged by the achievement of his students." ~Chauncey Veatch, America's Teacher of the Year, 2002

Body-

Excess weight makes your heart work harder. This extra strain can lead to hypertension, while losing weight lightens your cardiovascular workload. Strive to lose just 10 percent of your body weight to improve your heart health.

Spirit-

"Jesus said, 'Give, and it will be given to you. A good measure, pressed down, shaken together, running over, will be poured into your lap. For the measure you use, it will be measured to you." ~Luke 6:38

August 10:

Mind-

"Success is the culmination of failures, mistakes, false starts, confusion and the determination to keep going anyway." ~Nick Gleason, founder of CitySoft

Body-

By using self-control rather than deprivation a person can cut calories and still eat their favorite foods. Look for ways to save calories by comparing brands and flavors. For example, a slice of pepper jack cheese has seventy calories compared to mozzarella having a mere fifty.

Spirit-

Everything in this life is intricately interconnected to everything else, and each action you take, every word you say, alters the next moment that follows.

August 11:

Mind-

I am calm and cool and surrounded by healing energy.

Body-

The more fiber you eat, the fewer calories you absorb from all the other stuff you put in your mouth. Experts suggest getting twenty to thirty-five grams of fiber a day. If you are not eating that much now (and chances are you aren't, as most people get only ten to fifteen grams a day), work slowly up to that amount to minimize any discomfort from your digestive system. Fiber cannot do its job without it so drink at least eight, eight-ounce glasses a day. Track your fiber intake today to see how you are doing.

Spirit-

When God forgives our sin, it is gone forever.

August 12:

Mind-

Work should be and can be productive and rewarding, meaningful and maturing, enriching, and fulfilling, healing and joyful.

Body-

Imbibing a cool and nutritious smoothie can be good medicine. You can literally reverse nutrient deficiencies, slow down the oxidative processes (Aging) of your cells, make your nails stronger, make your hair shinier, protect yourself from heart disease and cancer, provide your body with the nutrients it needs to have more energy, and boost your metabolism for optimal fat burning.

Spirit-

To be almost saved is to be totally lost.

August 13:

Mind-

"Forget about all the reasons why something may not work. You only need to find one good reason why it will." ~Dr. Robert Anthony

Body-

Coffee has some health benefits, but lowering blood pressure isn't one of them. Caffeine can cause short-term spikes in blood pressure, even in people without hypertension. Drinking more than five hundred to six hundred milligrams of caffeine per day is associated with digestive problems, irregular heartbeats, muscle tremors, restlessness, and insomnia.

Spirit-

"Every calling is great when greatly pursued."
~Oliver Wendell Holmes

August 14:

Mind-

"What really scares me most, more than nukes or cancer is a man or woman without a sense of humor." ~Sid Caesar, comedian

Body-

Fresh vegetables contain antioxidants that can help reduce inflammation. Fiber rich vegetables such as cabbage, cauliflower, broccoli, and brussels sprouts are some of the vegetables that are a rich source of antioxidants, and it has also been proven that these vegetables can lower the risk of cancer and cardiovascular diseases.

Spirit-

"God doesn't look at how much we do, but with how much love we do it." ~Mother Teresa

August 15:

Mind-

"Finish each day and be done with it. You have done what you could; some blunders and absurdities have crept in; forget them as soon as you can. Tomorrow is a new day; you shall begin it serenely and with too high spirit to be encumbered with your old nonsense.

Body-

After a land workout, swimming a few laps can help you cool down, move blood through your muscles to help them recover, and help you relax as you glide through the water. Remember that swimming is a great cross training exercise for runners.

Spirit-

"When you judge another, you do not define them; you define yourself." ~Wayne Dyer

August 16:

Mind-

"I try to end each day saying, 'I am glad I did,' rather than, 'I wish I had.'" ~Barbara J. McMorrow

Body-

Plums are a very good source of vitamin C, which can help with iron absorption. They are also a good source of vitamin A, vitamin B2, and potassium. In addition, plums are a good source of dietary fiber. Additionally, both plums and prunes are full of phenols, natural compounds found in plants, which have protective properties. Plums also aid in hydration and fiber needs.

Spirit-

"There is no way to happiness; happiness is the way." ~Buddha

August 17:

Mind-

"Each friend represents a world in us, a world possibly not born until they arrive, and it is only by this meeting that a new world is born."
~Anais Nin, author

Body-

Adopting a healthful diet based on minimally processed fruits, vegetables, and whole grains promotes proper digestion and elimination that dramatically reduces the level of antigens and endotoxins in the bowel and blood.

Spirit-

"The Lord watches over you-the Lord is your shade at your right hand." ~Psalm 121:5

August 18:

Mind-

Achieving goals, whatever goals you set for yourself, can bring a satisfaction that is its own reward.

Body-

While there is no such thing as the "fountain of youth", there are many foods that can help combat the consequence of normal aging, such as sagging skin. Various berries may help counter the effects of aging on the surface of the skin. Try eating plenty of dark-skinned fruits, such as blueberries, blackberries, raspberries, cranberries, cherries, and grapes as these typically contain a higher concentration of antioxidants.

Spirit-

In frustrating times, remember that God is always up to something good.

August 19:

Mind-

"Pessimists need a kick in the can'ts." ~Mary Katherine and David Compton, authors

Body-

Turn down pain with self-hypnosis. Next time you are going to the dentist, or you have a pounding headache, lie down in a quiet spot, close your eyes, and breathe deeply. Imagine that you are at the top of a flight of ten stairs. Slowly walk down them, feeling each step under your feet, as you count backward from ten. When you reach the bottom, you should feel deeply relaxed, and your subconscious will be more receptive to your suggestions.

Spirit-

Reading the Bible offers us truth and strength.

August 20:

Mind-

Dwelling on negative thoughts holds you back from making new beginnings.

Body-

Improving your running form can help you run faster, more efficiently, and with less stress on your body and reduced the risk of injury. Your eyes should be focused on the ground about ten to twenty feet ahead of you. Keep your hands at your waist. As you run, keep your arms and hands as relaxed as possible. Don't clench your fists because it can lead to tightness in your arms, shoulders, and neck.

Spirit-

Even the person with little can give much to God.

August 21:

Mind-

Yes, you can! The power of positive thinking can change and improve your life. Maintaining positive thinking and attitude will drive you to success and happiness.

Body-

Beets help dilate blood vessels, which improves blood flow throughout the body. They are also packed with iron, which helps deliver oxygen throughout the body and wards off anemia. Anemia is a medical condition in which the red blood cell count or hemoglobin is less than normal. Any process that can disrupt the normal life span of a red blood cell may cause anemia. The normal life span of a red blood cell is typically around 120 days.

Spirit-

"Wait for the Lord; be strong and take heart and wait for the Lord." ~Psalm 27:14

August 22:

Mind-

Even small things can have a big impact on results.

Body-

Getting plenty of calcium and vitamin D can decrease your risk of developing a stress fracture by 20 percent. Your bone-healthy diet should consist of the following calcium-rich foods: milk, yogurt, cheese, vegetables, nuts, fish, breads, grains, and fruit. While you are planning your calcium rich diet, don't forget to include soy products.

Spirit-

"Love is good will towards others. Love is concern for others. Love wants good things to happen to others, even your enemies."

~Rev. Richard Taylor

August 23:

Mind-

"A smile is the closest distance between two people." ~Victor Borge

Body-

Bike riding is inherently relaxing, but the way you breathe can enhance the beneficial effects. Deep diaphragm breathing fully inflates your lungs while using less energy. Let your belly relax and drop toward your top tube (rather than raising your ribs). This calms you by maximizing inhalation and decreasing energy use.

Spirit-

Your task is not to seek love, but merely to seek and find all the barriers within yourself that you have built against it.

August 24:

Mind-

"Remember that no time is ever wasted that makes two people better friends." ~H. Jackson Brown Jr., author

Body-

Moving outside your comfort zone can help you make gains in speed and stamina. That can increase motivation and confidence and make running feel fun again. The challenge can be anything outside your comfort zone to include course, distance, terrain, even a different running partner. You can also add a cross training sport for a change of pace.

Spirit-

Delighting in the Lord can lead us from boredom to adventure.

August 25:

Mind-

All of life is a journey. Which paths we take, what we look back on, and what we look forward to is up to us. We determine our destination, what kind of road we will take to get there, and how happy we are when we get there.

Body-

Some experts have attributed the athletic advantage many cyclists and runners receive from a gluten-free diet to the fact that they're eating fewer high-glycemic (blood sugar spiking) foods, such as bagels, and pretzels, and more low-glycemic (blood sugar balancing) carbohydrates, such as fruits, non-starchy vegetables, and beans.

Spirit-

Every single thing in our lives can be used to serve God.

August 26:

Mind-

"A friend is a present you give to yourself."
~Robert Louis Stevenson, author

Body-

Making aromatherapy pillows is easy and cost effective. Aromatherapy pillows are good for relieving sore muscles and a stiff back of neck. Heat one for one or two minutes in the microwave for a hot pack that will loosen tight muscles or place one in the freezer to be used as a cold pack to relieve swelling.

Spirit-

Baptism does not remove our tendencies to sin but gives us access to the helping grace of God called "actual grace."

August 27:

Mind-

"Know this, someday all your challenges will make total sense to you." ~Karen Salmansohn

Body-

Any guilt about food, shame about the body, or judgement about health are considered stressors by the brain and are immediately turned into their electrochemical equivalents in the body. You could eat the healthiest meal on the planet, but if you are thinking toxic thoughts the digestion of your food goes down and your fat storage metabolism goes up. Likewise, you could be eating a nutritionally challenging meal, but if your head and heart are in the right place, the nutritive power of your food will be increased.

Spirit-

God does not call the prepared; God prepares the called.

August 28:

Mind-

There are four ways to move more:

1. Start early and go long.
2. Exceed expectations.
3. Have a sense of urgency.
4. Be resourceful and resilient.

Body-

On long bike rides, it is easy to lose track of how much time has passed since you last ate or drank. One easy solution is to set a timer on your watch, smart phone, or bike computer to go off at regular intervals. This can remind you to hydrate and fuel up as well as help train you to reach for your bottle or snack more regularly.

Spirit-

"Compassion is love in the face of suffering."

~Joseph Bailey, author

August 29:

Mind-

"Love is the purpose, the way and answer. You deserve love-everyone does." ~Andrea Hurst and Beth Wilson, authors

Body-

Well-rested athletes are typically 20 percent quicker at performing physical tasks than those who lack adequate rest. You need 7.5 to 8.5 hours of sleep on a regular schedule. The benefits include: more blood going to your liver to detoxify and more deep, slow wave restorative sleep during which we experience the highest levels of plasma growth hormone, which repairs soft tissue.

Spirit-

"True intelligence operates silently. Stillness is where creativity and solutions to problems are found." ~ Eckhart Tolle

August 30:

Mind-

"Successful people don't have any fewer problems than unsuccessful people; they just have a different mindset in dealing with them." ~John C. Maxwell, author, and motivational speaker

Body-

Bananas are full of potassium and magnesium, which both help to relax your muscles to give you a peaceful night's sleep. Bananas also have the added benefit of helping to lower your blood pressure while you sleep.

Spirit-

God has unlimited anytime minutes.

August 31:

Mind-

"When we leap, we must leap as though the net will appear. A leap in life, however big or small, is an act of commitment with the expectation of success." ~John O'Hurley, actor

Body-

Spending time in a group workout, whether water aerobics or swimming practice, is a great social outlet. Exchanging stories, challenging each other, and sharing in the hard work make swimming with others a rewarding experience.

Spirit-

None of us is worthy to approach God, but each of us is welcome.

September 1:

Mind-

"Two persons cannot long be friends if they cannot forgive each other's little failings."

~Jean de La Brutere, essayist, and moralist

Body-

Many people find that once they observe and release their negative mind-chatter about exercising, they have more energy, endurance and a welcome lightness of body and being. For extra credit this week, choose a new way to move your body.

Spirit-

There is a God-shaped hole inside every one of us, and we cannot buy something across the counter to fill that hole. The only thing that is going to fill that craving is God Himself.

September 2:

Mind-

"Your assumptions are your windows on the world. Scrub them off every once in a while, or the light won't come in." ~Alan Alda, actor

Body-

Getting fewer than three servings of fruit and vegetables a day can eat away at your health. Nutritional powerhouses filled with fiber and vitamins, fruits, and veggies can lower your risk of heart disease by 76 percent and may even play a role in decreasing your risk of breast cancer.

Spirit-

We need to understand that when God does not move in our circumstances, or when He does not move as quickly as we would like for Him to move, He may be waiting on purpose.

September 3:

Mind-

Everyone falls down. What matters is how you get back up.

Body-

During a rugged part of a bike ride, try counting pedal strokes. First count three to five strokes on your right leg. This creates the illusion that the left leg isn't working as hard. Then do the same with your left, and then five pedal strokes with focusing on either leg. Repeat until you have moved into an easier part of the ride.

Spirit-

God is more constant and connected to us than our shadow is.

Mind-

Creativity takes many forms-from writing, dancing, or painting to making dinner or planning a celebration for a friend. The only requirement is that we truly engage with the activity and in so doing, touch and express our deeper selves.

Body-

Many swimmers find an indirect benefit from swimming. They develop life skills such as sportsmanship, time management, self-discipline, goal setting, and an increased sense of self-worth through their participation in the sport.

Spirit-

Pride seems to keep a lot of people away from Christ and His fulness. The devil appeals to your selfish ambitions and your pride.

September 5:

Mind-

It is intimidating to shoot straight for major goals, so create sub-goals that will help get you to your ultimate goal.

Body-

Research shows that you are at greater risk of heart disease without a strong network of friends and family. Loneliness can cause inflammation, and in otherwise healthy people, it can be just as dangerous as having high cholesterol or even smoking.

Spirit-

When we cry, God shares our tears and our pain.

September 6:

Mind-

I stir up the gifts within me and use them to face all challenges. I am a real winner.

Body-

"If anything is sacred, the human body is sacred." ~Walt Whitman

Spirit-

"With wings of faith, you can rise and soar." ~Angela Maartinez

September 7:

Mind-

"If the essence of my being has caused a smile to have appeared upon your face or a touch of joy within your heart, then in living, I have made my mark." ~Thomas L. Odem Jr.

Body-

Many people use anxiety and stress to motivate themselves to lose weight. For example, "If I don't lose eight pounds for the party, I won't go," or "I'll never look good until I lose weight." This self-chosen stress feels energizing because it produces such alertness hormones as adrenaline; over time though, these fight-or-flight hormones can diminish metabolism.

Spirit-

"And we know that in all things God works for the good of those who love him, who have been called according to his purpose." ~Romans 8:28

September 8:

Mind-

Knowledge by itself is wasted on the unread.

Body-

When you do the same activity day after day, week after week, your mind isn't the only thing that gets bored-your muscles do too. To correct this, go for a hike on the weekend instead of doing your usual power walk. Find new strength moves that work the same muscles. Try a new type of exercise by slipping in a workout DVD.

Any little way to mix things up and challenge yourself with something new is a step in the right direction.

Spirit-

"Jesus said, "My yoke is easy, and my burden is light." ~Matthew 11:30

September 9:

Mind-

"When you realize how perfect everything is, you will tilt your head back and laugh at the sky." ~Buddha

Body-

Resistance training is aimed at developing power and strength. Most athletes include resistance training as an important component of their overall training plan. Resistance training increases muscle strength by pitting muscles against a weight, such as a dumbbell, barbell, or other type of resistance. A rubber band can even be used.

Spirit-

"John answered, "The man with two tunics should share with him who has none, and the one who has food should do the same." ~Luke 3:11

September 10:

Mind-

"Give people a bit of your heart rather than a piece of your mind." ~Helen Beam

Body-

Eating two eggs comprises 26 percent of your daily protein intake yet contains less than 10 percent of your recommended calories for the day. Thus, eggs can help you shed pounds. Hard-boiled eggs are fun to eat and easy to pack for

on-the-go lunches. Or mix chopped up hard-
boiled eggs with fresh lemon juice and olive oil,
leeks, dill, and salt and pepper to make a healthy
egg salad.

Spirit-

Following Christ is a choice we make every day.

September 11:

Mind-

"Hold a true friend with both hands." ~Nigerian
proverb

Body-

When the brain senses trouble with the food
supply, it does the simplest thing to conserve
energy. It will store fat and forget about building
muscle. Just the opposite of what you are trying

to do. Do not cut calories so much that you shut down your metabolism.

Spirit-

The Lord rejoices when we mature spiritually.

September 12:

Mind-

"Never underestimate the power of words to heal and reconcile relationships." ~H. Jackson Brown, Jr., author

Body-

Foods rich in vitamin D are essential for preserving muscle tissue. A 3.5-ounce serving of salmon contains almost 90 percent of the recommended daily allowance for vitamin D (600IU). Eat two 3.5 servings each week.

Spirit-

When we step outside our own concerns, we can help others with theirs.

September 13:

Mind-

Three small rules for living a happy life:

1. Start each day with a grateful heart.
2. Focus on the positive aspects of every person you encounter.
3. End each day with a grateful heart.

~Lucy MacDonald

Body-

According to traditional Chinese medicine (TCM), the whole of creation springs from the marriage of two opposite principles, yin and yang. Earth and sky, winter and summer, night, and day, and cold and hot are manifestations of this dynamic. Establishing harmony between these opposites means health, good weather, and good fortune, while disharmony brings disease, disaster, and bad luck.

Spirit-

What you do comes from what you think.

September 14:

Mind-

"Say no to anything that is not a high-value use of your time and your life." ~Brian Tracy

Body-

A medium-size baked sweet potato, skin included, offers five grams of fiber and only 103 calories. It is also a nutrition powerhouse, providing eye-healthy vitamin A, vitamin C, and some potassium, vitamin E, iron, magnesium, and phytochemicals like beta-carotene and lutein.

Spirit-

"Faith is not simply patience that passively suffers until the storm is past. Rather, it is a spirit that bears things with blazing serene hope." ~Corazon Aquino, former president of the Philippines

September 15:

Mind-

"Love and kindness are never wasted. They always make a difference. They bless the one who receives them, and they bless you, the giver. ~Barbara DeAngelis, author

Body-

An organic diet that is high in fiber and antioxidants from lots of fresh fruits and vegetables will improve the body's natural detoxification system.

Spirit-

"Live in such a way that those who know you but don't know God will come to know God because they know you." ~Unknown

September 16:

Mind-

Change starts from within with help from above.

Body-

In the United Staes, obesity continues to rise unabated. 65 percent of adults, or those over eighteen years of age, are overweight or obese.

The concern is not just that we are going to be less attractive and that we will be in larger-size clothes, it's that the cost of obesity related diseases would go through the roof.

Spirit-

"For we walk by faith, not by sight." ~2 Corinthians 5:7

September 17:

Mind-

"Open your heart…Open it wide; someone is standing outside." ~Mary Engelbreit, artist, and illustrator

Body-

Squeeze in hills by incorporating them into easy runs. No climbs nearby? Run overpasses or bridges. Mixing hills and flats will help you learn to keep an even effort level on changing terrain.

Spirit-

"You can keep a faith only as you can keep a plant, by rooting it into your life and making it grow there." ~Phillips Brook

It takes thirty days to form a habit, forty-five days to make it a routine and ninety days to develop a lifestyle. Strive for a new lifestyle by making faith a regular part of your life.

September 18:

Mind-

"When you live your life with an appreciation of coincidences and their meanings, you connect with the underlying field of infinite possibilities." ~Deepak Chopra

Body-

Eating a gluten free diet that's higher in protein and lower on the glycemic scale enables the body to gradually learn to use energy more efficiently from fat stores and to be less dependent on the food in the stomach. Low glycemic foods digest more slowly, which allows you to feel fuller for longer.

Spirit-

Each one of us is beautiful, because each one of us is God's child.

September 19:

Mind-

Worrying about what will happen if you don't get there will only bog you down.

Body-

Potassium helps lower blood pressure by counteracting sodium's ill effects. People with high blood pressure, African American and people who are middle-aged or older should get no more than 1,500 milligrams of sodium each day and should meet the potassium recommendation through food. Potassium-containing food sources include leafy greens, such as spinach and collards, fruit from vines, such as grapes and blackberries, and root vegetables, such as carrots and potatoes.

Spirit-

The life given away in loving service to others is the most fulfilled.

September 20:

Mind-

You must understand how to love through the worst parts of life, so you never take the best parts for granted.

Body-

Top your salads with chia seeds as they contain the sleep-inducing amino acid tryptophan. The tryptophan in chia seeds, like in turkey, raises melatonin and serotonin levels, which promotes stable sleep. With more than twice the tryptophan of turkey, you will need just two ounces of chia seeds to help you sleep.

Spirit-

God gives us courage to act in the face of our fear.

September 21:

Mind-

"True greatness consists in being great in the little things." ~Charles Simmons

Body-

Have you ever noticed how most of the diet and nutrition books on the market have you counting protein grams, fat grams, carbohydrate grams, portions, calories, servings, and points? You would think you were consuming a bunch of numbers. It's as if eating is a sporting event where you keep score or a business transaction with the body where you track debits and credits.

Spirit-

It is well for us to remind ourselves that if Jesus is not the center of our lives, we are self-centered.

September 22:

Mind-

"The future is literally in our hand to mold as we like. But we cannot wait until tomorrow. Tomorrow is now." ~Eleanor Roosevelt

Body-

By following current guidelines on exercise
(thirty minutes a day, most days a week), you
can bring down your blood pressure
significantly.

Spirit-

"We are therefor Christ's ambassadors, as
though God were making his appeal through us.
We implore you on Christ's behalf: Be reconciled
to God." ~2 Corinthians 5:20

September 23:

Mind-

Meditation, cleansing, self-analysis, exercise-it is
all focused on one goal: living your life in a fully
conscious way.

Body-

Drinking too much alcohol can elevate blood pressure in some people. A drink is defined as one twelve-ounce beer, one five-ounce glass of wine or one shot of liquor. The moderate consumption of alcohol appears to be more effective than most other lifestyle changes that are used to lower the risk of heart and other diseases.

Spirit-

"You can never cross the ocean unless you have the courage to lose sight of the shore."
~Christopher Columbus

September 24:

Mind-

"Only settle for your best; you'll be amazed at the results." ~Vince Lombardi

Body-

Some people find riding a roller coaster to be extremely stressful; others find it thrilling. It all depends on your perspective. People who have learned to identify and acknowledge stressful thoughts and think them through show notable improvements in their inner calm.

Spirit-

Even though you may be wrestling with a poor self-image, surely you can believe that you are more valuable than a bird and look how well your heavenly Father takes care of them.

September 25:

Mind-

"I can complain because rose bushes have thorns or rejoice because thorn bushes have roses. It's all how you look at it." ~J. Kenfield Morley

Body-

Popcorn with Parmesan cheese provides a delicious combination of carbohydrates and dairy. Dairy has tryptophan in it, which is a precursor to a sleep-inducing hormone, and the carbohydrates in the popcorn help your brain absorb tryptophan better. The standard serving for air-popped popcorn is a three-cup serving.

Spirit-

Trust God's ways: they work.

September 26:

Mind-

"The positive thinker sees the invisible, feels the intangible, and achieves the impossible." ~Unknown

Body-

Physical health and fitness can be achieved through a balance of endurance, flexibility, speed, and power. Endurance increases the strength of the heart and therefore its capacity to pump the blood that takes nourishment to the other organs of the body. Flexibility is achieved through stretching. Speed and power are developed through vigorous exercises like weightlifting or sprinting.

Spirit-

"Our beliefs about what we are and what we can be precisely determine what we can be." ~Tony Robbins

September 27:

Mind-

"Perseverance is not a long race. It is many short races one after another." ~Walter Elliott

Body-

Broccoli, a member of the cabbage family, is rich in iron, which carries oxygen to muscles, giving them energy. Sauté this dark green vegetable and then add lemon juice; the acid content helps speed iron absorption. Eat one to two cups of broccoli each week.

Spirit-

"Ordinary people believe only in the possible. Extraordinary people visualize not what is possible or probable, but rather what is impossible. And by visualizing the impossible, they begin to see it as possible." ~Cherie Carter-Scott

September 28:

Mind-

"Courage doesn't always roar. Sometimes courage is the quiet voice at the end of the day saying, 'I will try again tomorrow.'"

~Mary Anne Radmache

Body-

To optimize the power of a healthy diet, perform just twenty to thirty minutes of weight-bearing exercise several times a week. Weight-bearing exercise is essential for building and maintaining healthy bones.

Spirit-

"On the mountains of truth, you can never climb in vain; either you will reach a point higher up today, or you will be training your powers so that you will be able to climb higher tomorrow."
~Friedrich Nietzsche

September 29:

Mind-

"There is the risk you cannot afford to take, and there is the risk you cannot afford *not* to take."
~Peter Drucker

Body-

Your body needs fuel to start the day, and when it's deprived of food for longer than twelve hours, your metabolic rate can lower by 40 percent. When you skip breakfast, your body recognizes that you're not eating normally, so it cuts your metabolism down.

Spirit-

"If God be for us, who can be against us?"
~Romans 8:31

September 30:

Mind-

"Nothing gives one person so much advantage over another as to remain always cool and unruffled under all circumstance." ~Thomas Jefferson

Body-

Getting less than six hours of sleep a night dramatically increases your risk of high blood pressure. When we sleep well, we wake up feeling refreshed and alert for our daily activities. Sleep affects how we look, feel, and perform in a daily basis, and can have a major impact on our overall quality of life.

Spirit-

"My times are in your hands; deliver me from my enemies and from those who pursue me." ~Psalm 31:15

October 1:

Mind-

"Life is 10 percent of what happens to me and 90 percent of how I react to it." ~Charles Swindoll

Body-

To improve your blood flow, don't just stand there waiting for the microwave to beep. Launch into a turbocharged set of jumping jacks. Or put the phone on speaker when you are holding for customer service and de-agitate with the same jumping jacks.

Spirit-

"May the God of hope fill you with all joy and peace as you trust in him, so that you may overflow with hope by the power of the Holy Spirit." ~Romans 15:13

October 2:

Mind-

"The only way to be a friend is to be one."
~Ralph Waldo Emerson

Body-

Eating excess sugar destroys collagen, subsequently causing facial wrinkles. To help cut down on sugar, eliminate hidden glucose "spikers" often consumed at breakfast time-fruit-flavored yogurt and ketchup. Instead, decide on a whole-grain bagel with ow-fat cream cheese spread and a fresh orange. Remember, fresh fruit has more fiber and less calories than orange juice.

Spirit-

God is the ultimate and only steady source of renewal.

October 3:

Mind-

"Friendship improves happiness and abates misery by doubling our joys and dividing our grief." ~Joseph Addison, essayist, and poet

Body-

Nutrient-dense whole grains-such as buckwheat, quinoa, and brown rice-provide complex carbs, fiber, iron, and B vitamins. These foods tend to make us feel fuller longer, therefore stopping us from eating more calories.

Spirit-

"Therefore encourage one another and build each other up, just as in fact you are doing." ~1 Thessalonians 5:11

October 4:

Mind-

I am calm. I have peace of mind. There's happiness in my heart.

Body-

People use an average of 50 percent body language to 50 percent verbal language when communicating. If you cannot pick up the subtle nuances of the body language someone is giving, the message you may be receiving verbally could be quite different than what they intended on it being. The more you try to use and learn how to pick up on body language signals the better you will get at it.

Spirit-

Regular spiritual nourishment gives us a fuller life in Christ.

October 5:

Mind-

"Use your talent (everybody has one) in any way you can. Don't keep it for yourself like a miser- spend it like a millionaire." ~Lucy MacDonald

Body-

Stains on teeth is a very common dental problem that has more to do with appearance rather than health. To remove stains from your teeth, rinse with a small capful of hydrogen peroxide. (Don't swallow it.)

Spirit-

By counting our blessings, we become more aware of them.

October 6:

Mind-

I let go of all the pressures of the day in exchange for a good night's sleep.

Body-

Whole grains benefit your entire body-they're helpful in protecting against cancer, cardiovascular disease, diabetes, and obesity-yet most of us don't get the recommended three one-ounce servings of whole grains each day. Enjoy a slice of whole-wheat toast for breakfast, a multi-grain roll with your salad at lunch and a plate of spaghetti for dinner.

Spirit-

"There are only two ways to live your life. One is as though nothing is a miracle. The other is as though everything is a miracle." ~Albert Einstein

October 7:

Mind-

"There isn't a person anywhere who isn't capable of doing more than he thinks he can." ~Henry Ford

Body-

Losing weight isn't about not eating. It's about regularly eating foods that are filling and rich I nutrients. When you don't eat enough, your metabolism slows, and your body senses deprivation and starts an emergency supply of calories you do consume. It's all about the balance.

Spirit-

"As the deer pants for streams of water, so my soul pants for you, O God." ~Psalm 42:1

October 8:

Mind-

"Help others get ahead. You will always stand taller with someone else on your shoulders." ~Bob Moawad, author, and motivational speaker

Body-

Doing many repetitions and sets of an exercise to build, shape, and define muscles beyond simply challenging them can produce a "burn" often viewed as a sign of achievement, but it isn't necessary. The "burn" could be due to running out of the calcium supply that is needed to keep muscles contracting.

Spirit-

"Do not store up for yourself treasures on earth, where moth and rust destroy, and where thieves break in and steal." ~Matthew 6:19

October 9:

Mind-

"Shared joys rather than shared sufferings make a friend." ~Friedrich Nietzsche

Body-

If you want to maximize metabolism, breathing is one of the most effective tools because the greater your capacity to take in oxygen, the higher your metabolic "burning power" will be. Breathe in more oxygen and you burn food more fully. Breathing more if you eat a lot is the same as exercising more if you eat a lot. The moral of the story? Breathe!

Spirit-

"Jesus said, 'Therefore I tell you, do not worry about your life, what you will eat or drink; or about your body, what you will wear. Is not life more important than food, and the body more important than clothes?" ~Matthew 6:25

October 10:

Mind-

"Life is like a taxi. The meter just keeps ticking whether you are getting somewhere or just standing still." ~Lou Erickson

Body-

A medium apple contains four grams of fiber; a large apple has five. Apples also offer a bit of vitamin C and potassium. The apple meets one of the recommended daily servings of fruit and by eating the fresh apple rather than drinking a glass of apple juice you are consuming less calories. Way to go!

Spirit-

"Faith goes beyond reason. It goes beyond what you can see. But it is as real as anything you can touch or feel." ~Henry Cloud, author

October 11:

Mind-

"a strong positive attitude will create more miracles than any wonder drug." ~Patricia Neal

Body-

Button mushrooms are a rich source of CLA (conjugated linolenic acid), a good fat that actually helps to burn other fats off and increase lean body mass. Eat just half a cup every other day. You can add the mushrooms into your favorite pasta dish such as lasagna or spaghetti or put the mushrooms into your salad at lunch. Be creative with them.

Spirit-

"Consider it pure joy, my brothers, whenever you face trials of many kinds, because you know that the testing of your faith develops perseverance. ~James 1:2-3

October 12:

Mind-

"Shoot for the moon. Even if you miss, you'll land among the stars." ~Les Brown

Body-

High in polyunsaturated fats, pine nuts may help you burn calories at a higher rate even when you are not very active. Eat two tablespoons three times a week. Substitute pine nuts for almonds in your favorite recipe.

Spirit-

The secret of health for both mind and body is not to mourn for the past, not to worry about the future, or not to anticipate troubles, but to live in the present moment wisely and earnestly." ~Buddha

October 13:

Mind-

"The heart ages last." ~Sylvester Stallone, actor

Body-

Women in their fifties need to consume alternative sources of estrogen, like Phyto-estrogens, such as flaxseed. Consume thirty grams of flaxseed each day, which equals two teaspoons. Be sure to choose ground flaxseed for better absorption. Flaxseed can be added to oatmeal or eggs in the morning.

Spirit-

Today, God will give me what I need...and tomorrow God will do it again.

October 14:

Mind-

Little acts of kindness can add up to a lifetime of happiness.

Body-

A handful of walnuts contain almost twice as many antioxidants as an equivalent amount of any other commonly consumed nut. Stick to the handful in order to control calorie and fat intake.

Spirit-

Life truly is good if we choose to look for the good!

October 15:

Mind-

Pursuing a goal is a great way to get motivated and unlock your potential, as long as it's a target tailored to your abilities and ambitions.

Body-

Running hills are hard on your muscles, so refueling smartly will help speed recovery. Within thirty minutes of your run, eat a snack, like Greek yogurt topped with berries, which contains protein to repair muscles and antioxidants that can help fight soreness.

Spirit-

The fastest way to heaven is knee mail.

October 16:

Mind-

"Part of managing to grow old gracefully is that you just take the next step and hope you don't fall when you take it." ~Walter Cronkite, former CBS news anchor

Body-

Laughter has many benefits. It can stimulate many organs, enhance your intake of oxygen-rich air, stimulate your heart, lungs, and muscles, and increase the endorphins that are released by your brain. Laughter can also stimulate circulation and aid muscle relaxation, both of which can help reduce some of the physical symptoms of stress

Spirit-

"Love thy neighbor is a command, not a piece of advice." ~Bono, lead singer of U2

October 17:

Mind-

"In the end, nothing we do or say in this lifetime will matter as much as the way we have loved one another." ~Daphne Rose Kinga, author

Body-

Swap mild-tasting canola oil in place of less healthy fats, like butter and shortening, in place of less healthy fats, like butter and shortening, in recipes for quick breads and blueberry muffins.

Spirit-

"Keep your thoughts positive because your thoughts become your words. Keep your words positive because your words become your behaviors. Keep your behaviors positive because your behaviors become your habits. Keep your habits positive because your habits become your values. Keep your values positive because your values become your destiny.

October 18:

Mind-

"Let every man judge according to his own standards, by what he himself read, not by what others tell him." ~Albert Einstein

Body-

Rich in water content, watermelon keeps you feeling full and contains arginine, an amino acid that helps your body naturally burn calories. Watermelon is not only great as a delectable thirst-quencher, but it also helps quench the inflammation that contributes to conditions like asthma, diabetes, colon cancer and arthritis.

Spirit-

Nursing anger can poison our lives.

October 19:

Mind-

"If we fall, we don't need self-recrimination or blame or anger-we need a reawakening of our intention and a willingness to recommit, to be whole-hearted once again. ~Sharon Salzbar

Body-

Savor the zesty scent of an orange, and you could feel instantly relaxed. Orange essential oil is an ingredient commonly found in natural soap products to provide aroma to an everyday cleaning agent. The scent has a calming, anti-depressive effect.

Spirit-

Be Christlike in your relationships. Be kind and considerate to others.

October 20:

Mind-

"Life is not a matter of having good cards, but of playing a poor hand well." ~Robert Louis Stevenson

Body-

A person who can engage in light to moderate intensity physical activity, expanding about fifteen hundred calories per week, will most likely be able to lower the risk for coronary artery disease by about 25 to 50 percent. Invite a friend to stroll around the block with you.

Spirit-

"Train yourself to be godly." ~1 Timothy 4:7

October 21:

Mind-

"If you are distressed by anything external, the pain is not due to the thing itself, but to your estimate of it; and this you have the power to revoke at any moment." ~Marcus Aurelius

Body-

Your self-talk can make the difference between self-assurance and self-doubt, happiness and despair, success and failure. If you start making your self-talk more positive and affirming, and less defeatist and self-deprecating, your whole life will change for the better.

Spirit-

God doesn't judge us based on our looks; thankfully, He sees our hearts.

October 22:

Mind-

"Love makes the wildest spirit tame, and the tamest spirit wild." ~Alexis Delp

Body-

Every achievement, accomplishment, and success start, somewhere. Every task, large or small, begins with a first step. That first step can be hard to take. Yet one small step can lead to results you never imagined. Take the first step to a healthier, happier you. Decide on one thing you can accomplish today that puts you on the road to success.

Spirit-

When we obey and trust, God can use our small actions to accomplish much good.

October 23:

Mind-

"It is the mind that makes the body." ~Sojourner Truth

Body-

Self-esteem (Feeling good about yourself) is not something you are born with or that you automatically either have or don't have-it's something *you create.* And you *can* create it. Right now, right in the moment. Your self-image, your view of yourself and who you are is something you build every day. Start constructing now.

Spirit-

God's love has no limits.

October 24:

Mind-

"People take different roads seeking fulfillment and happiness. Just because they're not on your road doesn't mean they've gotten lost." ~H. Jackson Brown, Jr., author

Body-

Replace fruit-flavored yogurt with plain yogurt. Top this healthier treat with fresh berries or agave to naturally sweeten it. Instead of dousing your eggs with ketchup, try sriracha sauce made from chili peppers. It will give your eggs an extra kick and boost your metabolism as well. These are simple little changes that can have a big impact on your health.

Spirit-

Even when we don't know how to pray, God is near and responds to us.

October 25:

Mind-

"Don't let what you cannot do interfere with what you can do." ~John Wooden

Body-

"Some people, no matter how old they get, never lose their beauty. They merely move it from their faces into their hearts." ~Martin Buxbaum

Spirit-

My way to follow God may be uniquely different from other's paths.

October 26:

Mind-

Choose with no regret. Once you make a decision, go with it, and make it work for you.

Body-

Healthy carbs, such as quinoa, whole fruits, and whole wheat bread, provide a sustainable release of serotonin in the brain and have a high satiety value in the stomach, meaning they leave your stomach slowly and keep you fuller for a longer amount of time. This is good, fuller for longer equals less eating; less eating equals less calories.

Spirit-

"Faith can move mountains, but only if you lay down the shovel and stop trying to do it yourself." ~Amy Torkelson

October 27:

Mind-

"There is one quality that one must possess to win, and that is definiteness of purpose, the knowledge of what one wants, and a burning desire to possess it." ~Napolean Hill

Body-

Eating a snack between breakfast and lunch and then again between lunch and dinner keeps your metabolism elevated. Snacking will keep your energy even and your cravings almost nonexistent.

Spirit-

"Let there be justice for all. Let there be peace for all. Let there be work, bread, water, and salt for all. Let each know that for each the body, mind, and soul have been freed to fulfill themselves." ~Nelson Mandela

October 28:

Mind-

"If you are not using our smile, you're like someone with a million dollars in the bank and no checkbook." ~Les Giblin

Body-

"The resistance that you fight physically in the gym and the resistance that you fight in life can only build a strong character." ~Arnold Schwarzenegger

Spirit-

When you invite Christ into your heart, you can rely on Him to help you resist temptation.

October 29:

Mind-

"People become really quite remarkable when they start thinking that they can do things. When they believe in themselves, they have the first secret of success." ~Norman Vincent Peale

Body-

Cut the calories of your meal in half by swapping out one ingredient. Give macaroni and cheese a healthy makeover by using rice milk as a substitution for the milk and cream. Periodic small changes like this can save you calories overall.

Spirit-

Our faith rests on the foundation of God's love, spirit, and holiness.

October 30:

Mind-

"One of the things that my parents have taught me is never to listen to other people's expectations. You should live your own life and live up to your own expectations, and those are the only things I really care about." ~Tiger Woods

Body-

Muscles move more efficiently when they are toned, giving you a spring to your step. When a muscle is toned, the process is one of creating equilibrium. If muscles aren't exercised, they diminish. Toning is simply keeping the muscles you have already built in shape, while at the same time decreasing deposits of fat.

Spirit-

"Rejoice in the Lord always. I will say it again; Rejoice!" ~Philippians 4:4

October 31:

Mind-

"Act as if what you do makes a difference. It does." ~William James

Body-

No matter how healthy you eat, if you are eating too much, you will have a hard time maintaining a healthy weight. Remember portion control. The size of dinner plates has increased, making controlling your portions more difficult. You want half of your plate filled with veggies, a quarter filled with protein, and a quarter with carbohydrates (whole grains).

Spirit-

"When you step into the unknown, faith is knowing there will be something to stand on or you will be taught how to fly." ~Barbara J. Winter

November 1:

Mind-

Every journey begins with the first step.

Body-

Having sex regularly can add years to your life. An orgasm releases chemicals that make your skin glow, relax you and promote better sleep. Put sex on your calendar this week and keep the appointment no matter what. For more benefits, aim for two to three times a week.

Spirit-

"Probably the most important thing in the Bible is 'Love your enemies, do good to those who hate you.' This is what, to me, is the essence of Christianity." ~Dave Brubeck, jazz musician

November 2:

Mind-

"If a man does not keep pace with his companions, perhaps it is because he hears a different drummer." ~Henry David Thoreau

Body-

One reason you reach for cookies instead of carrots when you are in a bad mood is that your brain has been taught that dessert makes you feel better. As you start to develop healthy habits, you need to reinforce the message that going for a walk or eating fresh veggies is now the thing that gives you pleasure. Reset your dopamine levels.

Spirit-

"The wind blows wherever it pleases. You hear its sound, but you cannot tell where it comes from or where it is going. So, it is with everyone born of the spirit." ~John 3:8

November 3:

Mind-

"Everyone has problems and learning to share them is essential. Hiding pain requires an enormous amount of energy; sharing it is liberating." ~Carly Simon, singer, and songwriter

Body-

When you respond to someone else's good news in a super enthusiastic way, you spread that positive energy to yourself as well.

Spirit-

"Let us run with perseverance the race marked out for us." ~Hebrew 12:1-2

November 4:

Mind-

"Standing up for your beliefs builds self-confidence and self-esteem." ~Oprah Winfrey

Body-

A turkey burger with spinach on a whole-wheat bun is the perfect meal for restful sleep. You can thank the tryptophan in turkey for that.

Spirit-

Dreams can come true with commitment, hard work, and sacrifice. Dreams don't just happen; we need to do our part.
Dare to do something for God you've never done before.
Read about other cultures and pray for them.
Ask God to show you if you can "give" or "go".
Explore short-term church missions or trips to needy areas such as inner cities or places abroad.
Ask your pastor to put you to work. Ask him, "What needs doing around here?"
Make a promise to God to fulfill at least one dream a year.

November 5:

Mind-

"Be thankful for what you have; you'll end up having more. If you concentrate on what you don't have, you will never, ever have enough."
~Oprah Winfrey

Body-

Once cup of spaghetti squash, whose edible interior breaks up into noodle-like strands when cooked, has just forty-two calories with two grams of fiber. Spaghetti squash has a low-fat content and no cholesterol but is full of vitamins and minerals. Cooking spaghetti squash is very easy to prepare. You can boil, bake, or roast it.

Spirit-

Believe in miracles!

November 6:

Mind-

"Opportunity dances with those already on the dance floor." ~H. Jackson Brown, Jr., author

Body-

Chicken soup cures a cold because it slows immune cells down, reducing the inflammation that causes cold symptoms. Steam also helps clear stuffed airways.

Spirit-

"Love never fails." ~I Corinthians 13:8

November 7:

Mind-

"Nothing is more important than reconnecting with your bliss. Nothing is as rich. Nothing is more real." ~Deepak Chopra

Body-

Consistent lack of sleep can lead to a variety of health problems, including toxic build up, weight gain and aging, depression, irritability, and impatience, low sex drive, memory loss, lethargy, relationship problems, and accidents. Studies show that driving on only six hours of sleep is like driving drunk.

Spirit-

"Set you mind on things above, not on earthly things." ~Colossians 3:2

November 8:

Mind-

Live your life!

Body-

Wheat germ sprinkled on yogurt or cereal will provide you with a boost of vitamin B6, used in sleep aids for its ability to alleviate stress and anxiety. Try one teaspoon of wheat germ for a more restful sleep.

Spirit-

A sense of God's presence can sustain us through life's darkest nights.

November 9:

Mind-

Some scientists theorize that hypnosis bypasses your conscious thoughts and goes directly to your unconscious mind, while others believe that it helps you change the way you perceive the world.

Body-

To beat bloat, limit the amount of processed and prepared foods you eat.

Spirit-

"There is nothing that happens by chance in our universe. Everything unfolds according to higher laws-everything is regulated by divine order."
~Peace Pilgrim

November 10:

Mind-

"A journey of a thousand miles must begin with a single step." ~Lao Tsu

Body-

Simple swaps like replacing your shower curtain, your bedding, and the litter in your cat's box can make your home a much healthier place.

Spirit-

As precious a life on earth is, it doesn't compare to life with God in heaven.

November 11:

Mind-

The journey of life is easier because of God's light shining through friends and family.

Body-

Portion out larger homemade meals into handy leftover containers for your family to take to work and school, and prepare more dinners at home, rather than eating at restaurants or takeout. Brown bag lunches are lighter on calories as well as the pocketbook.

Spirit-

"Make a gift of your life and lift all mankind by being kind, considerate, forgiving, and compassionate at all times, in all places, and under all conditions, with everyone as well as yourself. This is the greatest gift anyone can give." ~David R. Hawkins

November 12:

Mind-

"Don't dream; work hard." ~Vince Lombardi

Body-

Massaging a healed scar a few minutes each day has been shown to flatten its fibers, so the scar looks and feels smoother.

Spirit-

"Pain is inevitable. Suffering is optional." ~Dalai Lama

November 13:

Mind-

Live as if this is all there is.

Body-

Sandalwood is valued in skincare for its moisturizing and skin-healing properties. Sandalwood is heavy, yellow, and fine-grained. Unlike other aromatic woods, sandalwood retains its fragrance for decades. Essential oils are extracted from the wood for use. Both the wood and the oil produce a distinctive fragrance that has been highly valued for centuries.

Spirit-

"The more we give love, the greater our capacity to do so." ~David R. Hawkins

November 14:

Mind-

Playfulness is a creative state. Watch a child play and see just how creative they are. Don't be shy, join in the fun.

Body-

Just a few minutes of stretching each day can help you stay limber for a lifetime. Improving flexibility means better balance, a straight back, less pain and fatigue, improved athletic performance, and even a clearer mind.

Spirit-

"Faith is the place between the way things are and the good that is sure to come." ~Brittany Kress

November 15:

Mind-

"I cannot always control what goes on outside. But I can always control what goes on inside." ~Wayne Dyer

Body-

Avoid fried foods. Choose grilled, steamed, broiled, or lightly sauteed foods instead. Animal fat, fried foods, and dairy products clog your arteries and are the major cause of most health problems, such as obesity. Cholesterol, heart conditions, and cancer. Use good fats like vegetable oils, cold pressed virgin olive oil, flaxseed oil, avocado oil, grape seed, and almond oil.

Spirit-

"Let the peace of Christ rule in your heart." ~Colossians 3:15

November 16:

Mind-

We are not responsible for how others act, only how we act, so act responsibly.

Body-

A diet low in B vitamins can cause mood swings and anxiety. An easy way to make sure you are getting your recommended daily allowance is to eat a bowl of fortified whole grain cereal with 1 percent milk and a sliced banana every morning.

Spirit-

"Everyone and everything around you is your teacher." ~Ken Keyes, Jr.

November 17:

Mind-

"The hardcore individual who persists in being mean can be eventually melted by love. ~Joyce Meyer

Body-

Foods that are rich in protein are naturally high in tyrosine, an amino acid that helps boost dopamine, the brain's feel-good chemical. Eat two servings of fish per week and an egg or some lentils every day to help keep a good mood from going bad.

Spirit-

"People only see what they are prepared to see." ~Ralph Waldo Emerson

November 18:

Mind-

"Happiness is like a butterfly; the more you chase it, the more it will elude you, but if you turn your attention to other things, it will come and sit softly on your shoulder." ~Henry David Thoreau

Body-

Shallow "chest breathing" invites problems by delivering less air per breath into the lungs. Less air per breath leads to a higher number of breaths, putting in motion a series of physiological changes that constrict blood vessels. Less oxygen reaches the brain, the heart, and the rest of the body as a result.

Spirit-

The Lord is waiting to forgive your sins the moment you turn to Him with all your heart.

November 19:

Mind-

"Nothing shows a man's character more than what he laughs at." ~Johann Wolfgang Von Goethe

Body-

Antioxidants and other nutrients in egg yolks help prevent macular degeneration, the leading cause of blindness in older adults; they also protect the retina from UV sun damage. Macular degeneration can make it difficult or impossible to read or recognize faces, although enough peripheral vision remains to allow ither activities of daily life.

Spirit-

"When a person really desires something, all the universe conspires to help that person realize his dream." ~Paulo Coelho

November 20:

Mind-

"Just for today, no matter where I am going, or what I am doing, or who I am doing it with, it is my intention to focus on the positive." ~Lucy MacDonald

Body-

If you are diagnosed with flu or another respiratory tract infection, your odds of having a heart attack are five times higher during the three days after diagnosis than it would otherwise. Infections can bring on an inflammatory response, which can trigger a heart attack or stroke. A flu vaccine may help protect against infection-induced heart stress.

Spirit-

At the end of life's journey, we will be greeted by our loving Savior.

November 21:

Mind-

"A friend is someone who knows you and loves you for what you were and who you are, and who also shares your hopes and dreams for who you can become." ~H. Jackson Brown, Jr., author

Body-

About 4 percent of adults have attention deficit hyperactivity (ADHD), and many others have never been diagnosed. A diagnosis can be important. Adults with ADHD tend to have lower incomes as well as higher rates of accidents, unplanned pregnancies, and substance abuse than those without it.

Spirit-

"The day, water, sun, moon, night-I do not have to purchase these things with money." ~Plautus

November 22:

Mind-

The only reason people get lost in thought is because it's unfamiliar territory.

Body-

To prevent overeating, drink two eight-ounce glasses of water before each meal. Water fills your stomach, making you feel full. So, reach for water before opening the fridge.

Spirit-

"Learn to get in touch with the silence within yourself and know that everything is this life has a purpose." ~Elisabeth Kubler-Ross

November 23:

Mind-

The more you become aware of the effects of each choice you make, the more you will be able to choose differently and better for yourself.

Body-

Brown rice is good for you, but black rice is even better. That's because the bran hull contains significantly higher amounts of vitamin E, which bolsters the immune system and protects cells from free radical damage. Black rice is a whole grain grown in Asia. It is high in fiber and nutrition, with a sweet nutty flavor that forms the base for exotic desserts and savory side dishes.

Spirit-

"Now faith is being sure of what we hope for and certain of what we do not see." ~Hebrew 11:1

November 24:

Mind-

Continue to learn. Challenge yourself to attend a conference, register for a class or learn a new hobby. Celebrate yourself and the success you have had this year.

Body-

Winter is the perfect time to dial back intensity. Don't worry about hitting a target pace or running a certain number of miles, just lay a foundation for the year.

Spirit-

"And as we let our own light shine, we unconsciously give other people permission to do the same." ~Nelson Mandela

November 25:

Mind-

Failure is not an option!

Body-

Eighty percent of people who lose weight and keep it off eat breakfast every day.

Spirit-

"A bird doesn't sing because it has an answer, it sings because it has a song." ~Maya Angelou

November 26:

Mind-

Add to your calendar an activity that better reflects what you want your priorities to be.

Body-

When we see flowers, our brain may instantly conjure festive memories. Put a vase of daisies on your kitchen table to start your morning right. Winter is right around the corner so why not bring a reminder of warmer climes inside to enjoy.

Spirit-

"Peace comes from within. Do not seek it without." ~Buddha

November 27:

Mind-

Surround yourself with positive influences. Always have access to positive people and resources.

Body-

The next time you throw out your back or do too many crunchies, hit a comedy club or watch old reruns. A good laugh significantly raises pain tolerance by flooding the brain with endorphins, natural opiates that are produced in the central nervous system and can dull your aches and pains as effectively as a pill.

Spirit-

"Joy is a net of love by which you can catch souls." ~Mother Teresa

November 28:

Mind-

Identify what you are looking to improve, change or accomplish. Do this first so you can establish a focal point.

Body-

The more motivational your tunes are, the quicker you move and the more calories you burn. Research shows that music tempo can increase your endurance by 15 percent. What are you waiting for? Pick up the tempo.

Spirit-

"Adopt the pace of nature; her secret is patience." ~Ralph Waldo Emerson

November 29:

Mind-

"In the middle of difficulty lies opportunity."
~Albert Einstein

Body-

Yellow has been called the color of optimism and joy. Consider a buttery hue for your walls or a rug or scatter a few pillows in a sunny shade on your couch.

Spirit-

"When I admire the wonders of a sunset or the beauty of the moon, my soul expands in the worship of the creator." ~Gandhi

November 30:

Mind-

Appreciate your friends. Invite them out to lunch and let them know how much you appreciate their friendship.

Body-

Nothing energizes like nature. Hang a large wall mirror opposite a window, and you will expand your view of sky, grass, and trees. The visual cues will stimulate you.

Spirit-

Prayer opens the door for God's power, and strength to fill us.

December 1:

Mind-

"Inspiration must come from within. If you have to look to others, you probably lack desire." ~Norm Duesterhoeft, captain, retired United States Army

Body-

To increase muscle mass, eat more protein, the building blocks of muscle. Roman beans are an excellent source, containing more protein than most other legumes. Eat two to three cups of these cooked beans each week.

Spirit-

"I am not a saint, unless you think of a saint as a sinner who keeps trying." ~Nelson Mandela

December 2:

Mind-

Do what you love.

Body-

The acetic acid found in balsamic vinegar helps activate genes that burn fat and increase satiety, so you feel fuller. Eat two tablespoons with meals, whenever possible, and mix with a little olive oil to replace other salad dressings.

Spirit-

"He is before all things, and in him all things hold together. ~Colossians 1:17

December 3:

Mind-

"Sometimes you have to let go to see if there was anything worth holding on to." ~Unknown

Body-

Women report sexual satisfaction increases with age, and arousal and orgasm are frequent, despite having low sexual desire. Women want to engage in sex for multiple reasons, including sustaining relationships even when the libido wanes late in life.

Spirit-

"All you need to do to receive guidance is to ask for it and then listen." ~Sanaya Roman

December 4:

Mind-

"Greatness lies not in being strong, but in the right use of strength. ~Henry Ward Beecher

Body-

Oranges contain a pharmacy's worth of salves for the heart. The soluble fiber pectin acts like a giant sponge, sopping up cholesterol in food and blocking its absorption, just like a class of drugs known as bile acid sequestrants. And the potassium in an orange helps counterbalance salt, keeping blood pressure under control.

Spirit-

The power of God is at work in people and places we wouldn't expect it to be.

December 5:

Mind-

"Satisfaction of one's curiosity is one of the greatest sources of happiness in life." ~Linus Pauling

Body-

Legumes (dried beans, such as kidney and garbanzo) are very high in potassium, as well as fiber and natural antioxidants that provide health benefits. This is the perfect time of the year to prepare a big pan of savory bean soup.

Spirit-

"Genuine beginnings begin within us, even when they are brought to our attention by external opportunities." ~William Bridges

December 6:

Mind-

"Always leave enough time in your life to do something that makes you happy, satisfied, even joyous. That has more of an effect on your economic well-being than any other single factor." ~Paul Hawken

Body-

The leafy greens of a spinach salad are packed with magnesium and help regulate your body's level of cortical, which tends to get depleted when you're under pressure. Remember to limit the amount of salad dressing you use to prevent calorie overload.

Spirit-

"The purpose of our lives is to be happy."

~Dalai Lama

December 7:

Mind-

Dreams will remain dreams until you give them a chance to become reality.

Body-

Learning how to satisfy your craving sensibly is a major part of sticking with a weight loss plan. When you are craving starch, try roasting peeled sweet potato cubes in a hot oven with a little olive oil and your favorite herbs, such as rosemary or oregano.

Spirit-

"When you dance, your purpose is not to get to a certain place on the floor. It's to enjoy each step along the way." ~Wayne Dyer

December 8:

Mind-

"When you come upon a path that brings benefit and happiness to all, follow this course as the moon journeys through the stars." ~Buddha

Body-

According to a new study, drinking six or more cups of coffee per day can lower a man's risk of fatal prostate cancer by up to 60 percent. Avoid the extra calories that cream, and sugar would add. Enjoy your coffee black.

Spirit-

"Don't worry about what you don't have if you do have faith." ~Rick Warren, pastor

December 9:

Mind-

"Be a warrior not a worrier. Create a list of all the times you've gotten things you didn't think were gettable. When faith is lagging, lug out this list." ~Karen Salmansohn, motivational speaker

Body-

If you feel like you live in your car, you probably consume a lot of calories there too. Maybe you wolf down snacks straight out of the bag, with little idea of how much you have inhaled, or you pull into the nearest drive-thru for a shake. Preempt unrestrained eating by packing portable, calorie-controlled nibbles such as small bags of cashews or an apple. Even half of a PB&J on whole wheat will do the trick.

Spirit-

"Be the change that you wish to see in the world." ~Gandhi

December 10:

Mind-

Companies don't exist in reality. They only exist on paper for legal purposes. In reality, companies are made up of entities called people.

Body-

Muscle grows or shrinks because training increases the size of muscle fibers, whereas detraining reduces their size. Fat cells have their own life, expanding when you eat too many calories and shrinking when you eat less. Finding the right balance is the key.

Spirit-

"People travel to wonder at the height of the mountains, at the huge waves of the seas, at the long course of the rivers, at the vast compass of the ocean, at the circular motion of the stars, and yet they pass by themselves without wondering." ~St. Augustine

December 11:

Mind-

You never know the full story of the person standing in front of you. Treat them as an angel in disguise because they just might be.

Body-

If you confine sweets to the end of the meal, you have all the built in protection to keep blood sugar on an even keel, avoid between-meal sweets at all costs-and when you do indulge, don't eat more than you can hold in the cup of your hand. But a few bites of candy after a meal will have little effect on your blood sugar and insulin-and can be quite satisfying.

Spirit-

"Happiness cannot be traveled to, owned, earned, worn, or consumed. Happiness is the spiritual experience of living every minute with love, grace, and gratitude." ~Denis Waitley

December 12:

Mind-

"You need to claim the events in your life to make yourself yours." ~Anne-Wilson Schaef

Body-

Start your meal with a salad. It soaks up starch and sugar. Soluble fiber from the pulp of the plants, such as beans, carrots, apples, and oranges, swells like a sponge in your intestines and traps starch and sugar in the niches between molecules. Soluble fiber eventually dissolves, releasing glucose. However, that takes time. The glucose it absorbs seeps into your bloodstream slowly, so your body needs less insulin to handle it.

Spirit-

"He who is filled with love is filled with God himself." ~St. Augustine

December 13:

Mind-

"It always comes back to the same necessity: go deep enough and there is a bedrock of truth, however hard." May Sarton

Body-

"Over the years your bodies become walking autobiographies, telling friends and strangers alike of the minor and major stresses of your life." ~Marilyn Ferguson

Spirit-

"If you judge people, you have no time to love them." ~Mother Teresa

December 14:

Mind-

"At the height of laughter, the universe is flung into a kaleidoscope of new possibilities. ~Jean Houston

Body-

Sprinkle these spices on your food for a lift that lingers. Cinnamon can stabilize your blood sugar, leading to sustained energy. Cumin may raise iron levels, and coriander can help calm by elevating levels of the nutrient magnesium, which gets depleted in times of stress.

Spirit-

"God is our refuge and strength, an ever-present help in trouble." Psalm 46:1

December 15:

Mind-

"Words are a form of action, capable of influencing change." ~Ingrid Bengis

Body-

"Champions aren't made in gyms. Champions are made from something they have deep inside them, a desire, a dream, a vision. They have to have the skill and the will. But the will must be stronger than the skill." ~Muhammad Ali

Spirit-

"Giving is the secret of a healthy life. Not necessarily money, but whatever a person has of encouragement, sympathy and understanding," ~John D. Rockefeller

December 16:

Mind-

"Make allowances for your friends' imperfections as readily as you do for your own." ~H. Jackson Brown, Jr., author

Body-

Don't let yourself fall into the trap of taking a long, luxurious nap on a weekend unless you have the flu or other illness. If you do, sleeping at night will become mission impossible. But if you have had a rough night of sleeplessness, a true catnap that lasts no more than twenty minutes.

Spirit-

"Pray that your loneliness may spur you into finding something to live for, great enough to die for." ~Dag Hammerskjold

December 17:

Mind-

"Courage is as often the outcome of despair as hope; in the one case we have nothing to lose, in the other, all to gain." ~Diane DePoiters

Body-

If you are looking to cut down on carbohydrates, your focus should be on the refined, mass-produced kind. Vegetables are fine. High-starch vegetables are also fine, just go easy on them. Fruits are also great-just be sure you focus on variety and don't limit your fruit to pineapple, grapes, bananas, and dried fruit, as these can be high in natural sugar. Whole grains such as brown rice are preferable to their white cousins.

Spirit-

God builds on the best in us.

December 18:

Mind-

"Don't let the fear of the time it will take to accomplish something stand in the way of your doing it. The time will pass anyway; we might just as well put that passing time to the best possible use." ~Earl Nightingale

Body-

Substitute canola oil for butter in breads and muffins. Canola contains the antioxidant vitamin E and heart-healthy monounsaturated fat.

Spirit-

"If someone listens, or stretches out a hand, or whispers a word of encouragement, or attempts to understand a lonely person, extraordinary things begin to happen." ~Loretta Girzartis

December 19:

Mind-

"You must take personal responsibility. You cannot change the circumstances, the seasons, or the wind, but you can change yourself. That is something you have charge of. You don't have charge of the constellations, but you do have charge of whether you read, develop new skills, and take new classes." ~Jim Rohn

Body-

A few drops of vanilla, orange, peppermint, or almond extract will boost the flavor of a smoothie with adding calories.

Spirit-

"The great awareness comes slowly, piece by piece. The path of spiritual growth is a path of lifelong learning. The experience of spiritual power is basically a joyful one." ~M. Scott Peck

December 20:

Mind-

"My life is my message." ~Mahatma Gandhi

Body-

Sodas are either full of sugar or artificial sweetener. When you want something sweet, try juices like peach and watermelon. Or have a piece of fruit like an apple or orange. These foods are naturally sweet and refreshing. Your body will appreciate the energy from these foods. As a coffee replacement use My Whey made out of goat's milk whey. It looks like and tastes like instant coffee. All you do is add hot water and you have instant energy, because it contains lots of minerals and protein.

Spirit-

"To us also, through every star, through every blade of grass, is not God made visible if we will open our minds and our eyes. ~Thomas Carlyle

December 21:

Mind-

Time is given to you today. You cannot keep it; you must spend it or invest it accordingly.

Body-

Between the office candy bowl, the vending machine, and a co-worker's homemade brownies, your office probably stocks more snacks than a 7-Eleven. And since you are only nibbling, the calories don't count, right? Wrong! Launch a counteroffensive by bringing in healthy snacks such as roasted almonds or dark chocolate. Knowing that these treats are tucked away will give you the strength to resist the disastrous jelly doughnuts.

Spirit-

"Trees are the earth's endless effort to speak to the listening heaven." ~Rabindranath Tagore

December 22:

Mind-

The door to happiness opens outward.

Body-

If you want to spoil yourself, splurge for some bamboo bedding. Bamboo feels silkier than even some sky-high-thread-count cotton sheets. It is hypoallergenic, and because it comes from an abundant plant, it's more sustainable. Look for 100 percent bamboo sets, not cotton. Buy a set, wrap it, and put it under the tree for yourself.

Spirit-

"A good man is not a perfect man; a good man is an honest man, faithful, and unhesitatingly responsive to the voice of God in his life."

~John Fischer

December 23:

Mind-

"Affirmations are like prescriptions for certain aspects of yourself you want to change." ~Jerry Frankhauser

Body-

Traditional Chinese Medicine (TCM) excels in using herbs for stress, energy, and overall wellness, and it all starts with ginseng root. Ginseng can be ingested directly as food and can be added like seasonings, or a major ingredient in several dishes, Root powder, root shavings, sliced roots, and even whole roots are used in soups and teas.

Spirit-

Father may my home be a place where others feel welcomed and loved. Most of all, God may my home be always open to you. Please live here with me. Amen

December 24:

Mind-

Fast talk means fast thinking, which automatically boosts your energy. Speed-talk your way through your next friendly chat and feel that breathless rush gives you a boost.

Body-

Having satisfying sex two to three times per week can add as many as three years to your life. Regular sex may also lower your blood pressure, improve your sleep, boost your immunity, and protect your heart.

Spirit-

"[I]in order that they may know the mystery of God, namely, Christ, in whom are hidden all the treasures of wisdom and knowledge."

~Colossians 2:2-3

December 25:

Mind-

True giving knows no season, requires no reason. It is for love.

Body-

Few sports and activities can claim to be a total body workout, but cross-country skiing is just that. It combines both a lower body and upper body workout, while simultaneously working both the "pulling" and "pushing" muscles of each region. Every major muscle group is involved in propelling the skier forward, and even muscles that don't seem to be in use are actively involved to balance and coordinate the entire body.

Spirit-

"If there is love in your heart, Christmas can last forever." ~Marion Schoeberlein

December 26:

Mind-

"Strange how no two snowflakes are alike, but yet they stick together." ~Dorothy Player

Body-

Ice-skating offers positive effects for your cardiovascular health. It is a low-impact exercise, so it is not as hard on your joints as running is. Ice-skating makes your heart muscles healthy, providing significant protection from coronary artery diseases and subsequent heart attacks. It also aids in weight loss as you can burn 250-810 calories per hour.

Spirit-

Will you let Him be your Savior now? He has loved you, loves you still. Ask Him now to forgive your sins and to hear you as you pray. He will. He has bought you with a great price, His own blood. He is seeking you now.

December 27:

Mind-

"Friends multiply blessings and divide burdens."
~Gail D. White

Body-

Snowshoeing is a great workout; However, snowshoeing will cause you to use a lot of fluids in the process. Make sure you stay hydrated so you will have enough energy for the long haul.

Spirit-

We can trust in God's presence and provision every day.

December 28:

Mind-

I'm proud of the choices I make. My reward is good health and joy.

Body-

Exercising outdoors is possible during the winter but it's easy to get dehydrated. Dehydration causes decreased blood volume, which makes us more susceptible to hypothermia and frostbite. It's important to drink water frequently.

Spirit-

"The fishermen know that the sea is dangerous and the storm terrible, but they have never found these dangers sufficient reasons for remaining ashore."

~Vincent van Gogh

December 29:

Mind-

Here it is the end of the year; our journey together is almost over. You have done well, stay the course and keep improving yourself. Begin by asking yourself this question, "How are you getting to a happier you?"

Body-

The Mediterranean diet is one of the world's healthiest. Those who follow it are less likely to develop high blood pressure, high cholesterol, or become obese. The Mediterranean diet emphasizes healthy fats, fruits, and vegetables.

Spirit-

God is more constant and connected to us than our shadow is.

December 30:

Mind-

Peace produces more peace.

Body-

Planning your workouts and writing them down afterward is a great way to chart your progress. Being able to look back on how far you have come-a faster pace, bigger weights-will inspire you to stick to it.

Spirit-

Sharing our faith can prepare others to receive God's grace.

December 31:

Mind-

Don't give up!

Body-

Aroma therapists use peppermint in treating asthma, nausea, colic, cramps, colds, fevers, fainting, and headaches.

Spirit-

Each one of us can take joy in what we do for God.

Bonus Material

During a sleepover at grandma's house, my oldest granddaughter made me aware of her happiness, as well as my own. She was two years old, had just awoken from her nap and she sat in her crib talking and laughing to herself while I listened outside the door. She was in such a good mood, and as a result, so was I. I decided right there and then that when I grow up, I want to be just like Claire; Happy! But then I got to thinking, why shouldn't she be happy. She was only two years old after all. She had nothing to be sad about. She was at grandma's house, she knows she is well loved and besides, grandma gives her lot of snacks. Still, it made me pause and think about my happiness and how I achieved it.

True joy and happiness are valuable. To be happy is relatively easy; just decide to be a happy person. Abraham Lincoln observed that most people, for most of the time, can choose how happy or stressed, how relaxed or troubled, how bright or dull their outlook would be. The choice is simple really, choose to be happy.

Happiness in life is one of the most important things people seek or should be seeking. True Happiness is hard to achieve, and some people search their entire life and never find it. But there are people that do find true happiness in their lives. Some of these people find it without any money or great success. Some people find happiness in life while they are homeless, broke, and alone.

Happiness is part of human nature-people from every background, even from the opposite ends of the Earth, are equally well acquainted with how it feels and can recognize it in each other. Happiness in life is easy to experience but almost impossible to hold onto and keep. Everyone (even yourself) has been happy for a moment or two. The secret is being able to recognize happiness in your life and hold on to that feeling and not make yourself miserable.

Happiness is an emotion, but it is greatly influenced by the choices you make. You can choose to be optimistic rather than pessimistic, hopeful rather than doubtful.

Sure, life will throw you some curve balls, but not one can steal your happiness.

Remember, it is the journey that should bring you happiness, not the destination. Thinking that when I get a better job, get healthier, find the right person, etc., then I will be happy. This is cutting yourself short. What if it takes you ten years? Will you want to wait that long to feel these wonderful feelings of happiness? No, of course not. Quit kidding yourself if you said yes. It is about having happy moments as often as you can. Don't wait for some big happy moment to set you off. Be happy now. Be happy you are alive and able to read this. Many people overlook the meaning of their life, and they get stuck in their daily grind to get to the next paycheck, then to the next vacation. If that is you, stop thinking that way, quit reading this and go for a walk.

Another technique to having happiness in life is to surround yourself with happy people and things. If you surround yourself with lots of drama and negativity you won't be able to realize your full happiness potential. Happiness in life isn't going to come on its own. In most cases you will have to work towards it.

A newspaper in England once asked this question of its readers, "Who are the happiest people on the earth?" The four prize-winning answers were:
- A little child building a sandcastle.

- A craftsman or artist whistling over a job well done.
- A mother, bathing her baby after a busy day.
- A doctor who has finished a difficult and dangerous operation that saved a human life.

The paper's editors were surprised to find virtually no one submitted kings, emperors, millionaires, or others of riches and rank as the happiest people on earth.

W. Beran Wolfe once said, "If you observe a happy man, you will find him building a boat, writing a symphony, educating his son, growing double dahlias in his garden, or looking for dinosaur eggs in the Gobi Desert. He will not be searching for happiness as if it were a collar button that has rolled under a radiator. He will not be striving for it as a goal in itself. He will have become aware that he is happy in the course of living life 24 crowded hours of the day."

Be so happy that when others look at you, they become happy too.

Defining Happiness

According to the dictionary, happiness means:

1. The quality or state of being happy.
2. Good fortune; pleasure; contentment; joy.

Happiness is thought of as the good life, freedom from suffering, flourishing, well-being, joy, prospective, and pleasure.

Its pursuit is enshrined as a fundamental right in the United States and occupies most of us. But what do we really know about happiness? Can we study it? Are we born with it? Can we make ourselves happier? Who is happy and who is not, and why? What makes us happy? Researchers are learning more and more about the answers to these questions.

Psychologists say yes, and that there are good reasons for doing so. Positive psychology is "the scientific study of the strengths and virtues that enable individuals and communities to thrive." These researchers' work includes studying strengths, positive emotions, resilience, and happiness. Their argument is that only studying psychological disorders gives us just part of the picture of mental health. We will learn more about well-being by studying our strengths and what makes us happy. The hope is that by better understanding human strengths, we can learn new ways to recover from or prevent disorders and may even learn to become happier.

Researchers also distinguish between the moment-by-moment feeling of happiness produced by positive emotions and how we describe our lives when we think about it. Regardless of whether you had a good day or not, do you describe your life as a happy one? Or describe yourself as a happy person?

Since happiness is so subjective, can it really be measured and studied scientifically? Researchers say yes. They believe that we can reliably and honestly self-report our state of happiness and increases and decrease happiness. After all, isn't our own perception of happiness what matters? And if we can report it, scientists can measure it.

The Generational Debate

Ask your parents or grandparents to define happiness and they will surely talk about love, friends, and family. Next, they will probably mention succeeding in their chosen career, owning a nice home, and having a solid nest egg.

But ask a Gen Y, and the definition of success and happiness may sound quite different. As journalist Hannah Seligson recently wrote of her peers in the Washingtonian, "Instead of a steady job, they want a meaningful one that serves a larger purpose or fulfills a personal passion. And instead of settling down with a spouse and mortgage, they want more years of freedom to chase career dreams and explore different paths before they must make tradeoffs.

For Millennials, things like climbing the corporate ladder, socking away money for a home, and building up retirement savings have one serious drawback; they take a lot of time. And experience shows, Millennials do not like to wait. Perhaps because so many of their parents showered them in self-esteem, or perhaps because they witnessed the horrors of 9/11 at a young age and learned that life can be too short, Millennials tend to have a carpe diem philosophy. They want it all, and they want it now.

Laughter, the Best Medicine

A healthy dose of humor can make a significant contribution to your overall health and well-being. Science is learning what common sense has shown us all along; laughter is wonderful medicine and an important aid to healing. It revitalizes and relieves tension. No matter what problems you face today, look for humor.

It's all in the Attitude

Set a tone of happiness for the day by smiling as soon as you wake up each morning. First, smile at God, saying in your heart, *Thank You for watching over me all night.* Second, smile at the remembrance of at least one good thing that happened the day before. Third, smile at the thought of all the opportunities and blessings that await you during the day. Fourth, smile at the thought that God will be present throughout the day to help you with every crisis, challenge, or obstacle. Fifth, smile at the very fact that you are alive and *smiling*. And since you will have so many smiles, be sure and give some away!

The Power of Relationships

Finding happiness in a relationship may seem pointless when that relationship is unhealthy. On the other hand, there is a way to make changes with yourself, that may help. Finding happiness in your relationship is easy of you are happy within yourself to begin with. What if you are not happy with yourself? How do you work on self-fulfillment while trying to fix a broken relationship? Isn't that selfish?

Think of your relationship as a recipe. When you mix healthy ingredients together, the result is a healthy and tasty dish. When one or both if the ingredients is spoiled, your culinary creation is spoiled as well. Likewise, a healthy relationship is created when both people are mentally healthy. By nurturing yourself, you are improving your relationship recipe. Therefore, self-improvement is not a selfish act, but one that strengthens your relationship.

Happiness in your relationship is a two-way street. While you are working on your own self-help, don't forget about your partner. If they lack self-esteem, take the time to reassure them of their self-worth. Let them know that you appreciate the things they do for you. Take the time to make them feel good about themselves. It is vital to know you are valued in a relationship. Even if you have been together a long time, it helps to verify your importance to each other occasionally.

Sometimes we get caught up in everyday life and forget about ourselves for a while. The bills must be paid. The chores must be done. We must make sure all is right with family and friends. When this happens, our own happiness and sense of self-worth sometimes fall by the wayside. What have you done for yourself lately? When you feel neglected due to stress of everyday living, it is hard to find happiness in your relationship. Take the time to nurture yourself and your relationship will profit from your inner happiness.

Happy Now, Sad Later (Situational Happiness)

Is the glass half full or half empty? This is the classic question that determines whether one is an optimist or a pessimist. The purpose of the question is to demonstrate that the situation may be seen in different ways depending on one's point of view and that there may be opportunity in the situation as well as trouble. This idiom is used to explain how people perceive events and objects. Perception is unique to every individual and is simply one's interpretation of reality.

Situational happiness is when we depend on external circumstances in order to provide us with joy and well-being. We crave our "external world" to be a certain way, and if we don't get it then we are left disappointed and unhappy. Those who learn to cultivate emotional independence (especially dedicated meditation practitioners like Buddhist monks), find out how to find happiness that is independent of these external conditions. Some of the most common things we become dependent on for happiness include:

- Excessive eating.
- Alcohol and drugs.
- Movies, TV, music, video games, the internet, and other entertainment.
- Sex.
- Shopping and consumerism.
- People.
- Pets.
- Wealth and money.
- Traditions and routine.

These are all desires that we can develop a near-addictive personality toward. Of course, someone can develop an addictive personality toward nearly anything, but of course that doesn't make any of these habits *necessarily* bad. Only when one can no longer exercise these habits in moderation, and we begin to depend on them to enjoy ourselves, do these habits turn into a problem. Then we are emotionally dependent on them to live a fulfilling life.

The idea that one's emotional state should be determined by events is pervasive; it's no coincidence that the words happen and happy share a common root. Almost every action life performs is designed to improve its external conditions: every amoeba wriggling up a chemical gradient, every car on the road driven by someone to somewhere they'd rather be. But letting today's events determine today's mood is problematic because circumstances are transient and so happiness dissolves when the circumstances change, as they inevitably do. Seeking refuge in the impermanent and the unreliable allows minute-by-minute events hijack your emotions, your mind, yourself. To the extent that your emotions drive your behavior, situational happiness reduces your authenticity, by expressing a conditional, contingent version of you, not the absolute, essential you.

Habitually happy people know how they like to feel. They like to feel good and on top of their game all the time. They like to be and try to be energized, up, happy, and enthusiastic all the time. They continually try to do their best, feel their best and be at their best. Try to become a habitually happy person to avoid situational happiness.

Spiritual Happiness

There have been countless research studies on spiritual wellbeing or just being happy, and all have shown that feeling good about yourself or everyday situations maintains or improves one's health. Everyone seems to have a different way of finding happiness. Some people find it in religion while others might find it in food, exercise, favorite hobbies, family, and friends.

A spiritually happy person is in tune with and accepting of themselves. They feel no need to impress anyone or to compete. They love themselves (not in an egotistical way) the way they are. With spiritual happiness, you are not waiting to be rich before you can be happy, or to find the right person to be happy, or to have more friends to be happy. You don't need to look different to be spiritually happy. With spiritual happiness, you can look at the world with realistic eyes—seeing, experiencing, and responding to all the muddled mess that life can sometimes seem to be. Yet, in the depths of your being, you will know a peacefulness and contentment that never fades, even while the world may be crashing down around you.

Different How?

Pleasure or Happiness?

We are a pleasure-seeking society. Most of us spend our energy seeking pleasure and avoiding pain. We hope that by doing this, we will feel happy. Yet happiness and joy seem to elude many people. The reason for this is because there is a huge difference between happiness and pleasure. Pleasure is a momentary feeling that comes from something external-a good meal, our stock options going up, making love, and so on.

Pleasure has to do with the positive experiences of our senses, and with good things happening. Pleasurable experiences can give us momentary feelings of happiness, but this happiness does not last long because it is dependent upon external events and experiences. We must keep having the good experiences-more food, more drugs or alcohol, more money, more sex, more things-in order to feel pleasure. As a result, many people become addicted to these external experiences, needing more and more to feel a short-lived feeling of happiness.

Happiness on the other hand is a state of mind. It reflects what is going on inside us. Many people go out to the bar or get together with this person or that person all to find happiness. The sad thing is that these people will never find it. That is as long as they keep looking outside of themselves.

Content or Happy?
The American Heritage Dictionary records the definition of the word content as "satisfied" whereas happiness (a derivative of the word happy) means:
  1.) Characterized by good fortune.
  2.) Having, showing, or marked by pleasure.
From these definitions, it appears that happiness is a state of mind or attitude that is induced by the presence of favorable circumstances. To be content (based upon the definition of satisfy) means "to gratify or fulfill a

need or desire." Hence, it represents a state of mind that is induced when a need or desire is fulfilled...not necessarily because of favorable circumstances.

To be happy denotes a state of being that relies on positive experiences to reinforce its existence. Hence, when difficult times occur, you can fall from the state of happiness into the state of fear, anger, depression, and chaos until the negative stimulus is eliminated. However, to be content denotes a state of mind that is not based upon positive or negative stimulation...it is a feeling akin to peace of mind. To be content means that one accepts all circumstances as part of the natural rhythm of life...the cosmic flow that contains both peaks and valleys.

Joy vs. Happy?

Both joy and happiness are positive and desirable emotions where a person has a feeling of being satisfied. These feelings are based on certain reasons, and the nature that causes that feeling can differ. Joy comes from the inner self of a person and is connected with the source of life within you. It is caused by something exceptional and satisfying. The source of joy is something or someone greatly appreciated or valued, and it is not only about oneself, but also about the contentment of those people whom you value the most.

Happiness is an emotion experienced when in a state of well-being. The state of well-being is characterized by motions ranging from contentment to intense joy. Happiness is simply the state of being happy. It may be caused by good fortune, luck, or various other pleasures that range from person to person. Happiness is a result of something that is outside of you and gained by observing or doing that particular thing. Social networks and human relationships are the most important correlation with happiness. Happiness spread through relationships like friends, siblings, partners, and neighbors.

Gratitude

Ten Ways to Get More Energy by Being Thankful
Anne Naylor, a personal motivation coach, author, and Huffington Post blogger, advises that we all carry a precious resource with us: thankfulness. No one can take it away. However, you can either enhance or diminish your awareness of it. Here, Anne offers 10 tips for becoming grateful-and energized in the process.

1. **Gratitude Journal**
    Keep a gratitude journal. At the end of each day, write five things you feel grateful for from the

day: a smile from a stranger, a hug from your child, an unexpected compliment, a good meal, a moment of laughter with a friend.

2. **Before Sleeping**

    Go to bed with a smile, thinking about all you appreciate in your life. Breathe deeply and relax as you do so.

3. **Gratitude Dance**

    Take a few minutes and begin your day with a gratitude dance. Start your day as you would intend it to be. If your energy is flagging during the day-do it again. It will probably make you laugh, and that will energize and refresh you.

4. **Appreciate Family, Friends, and Co-workers**

    Bring to mind those close to you whom you love, and how thankful you are that they are part of your life. Make a note in your journal of your special people and why you appreciate them.

5. **Express Appreciation**

    At home, work, or in your community, take a little time to communicate your appreciation to those you value in person, over the phone, by e-mail.

6. **Midday Break**
   Take a short walk and count your blessings, feeling grateful as you do so. You will come back inspired and enthusiastic for the afternoon.

7. **Blessings in Disguise**
   When you are going through a tough time, it is harder to feel grateful. However, when you do, the results can be amazing. When things are not going your way, or the way you had intended, declare them a "blessing in disguise" and be grateful for them. This simple shift in attitude will make you a winner, no matter what happens.

8. **Gratitude Gathering**
   Bring a group of friends together for a gratitude gathering and recount the things you are grateful for. Conclude with a celebratory potluck meal.

9. **Nature Walk**
   Take a walk in nature and notice the beauty around you. Beauty might be in something very simple like a leaf, a bird in flight, sunlight on dew, an elegant branch of a tree, the color of the sky, the crunch of gravel, or the softness of grass beneath your feet. Allow yourself to feel the beauty and your gratitude for it.

10. **Be Grateful for You**

Last but absolutely not least, take a moment to notice the goodness of your intent; the caring you express to others; the endeavors you take to be true to your ideals, even at difficult times. Be grateful for and bless your qualities and strengths. There is no one else quite like you. Honor and appreciate yourself.

To read more of Anne Naylor's writing, check out her blog at http://www.huffingtonpost.com/anne-naylor/

Practicing Gratitude in Everyday Life
Have you ever made a wish for happiness when blowing out your birthday candles? Instead of making a wish for what you don't have, or what you want, stop and think about what you do have and what you are grateful for. You will find yourself appreciating your home, even though it needs work; your significant other, even though he or she is lacking in any number of qualities; and your day-to-day life.

We all have moments in our lives that are cause for big celebrations and thank you-birthdays, graduations, holidays, a new baby being born, or a job promotion. It is easy to pull out Champagne, light the candles on the cake, and go all out in celebration. But it is embracing the joyful simplicities of every day and discovering their simple delights that are the essence of life. We need to find joy, to be thankful for the everyday moments that bring us comfort and well-being.

All it takes is a shift in our thinking, a mindfulness to focus on what makes us glad to be alive. So, the next time you are driving, your mind full of tasks, look at the people strolling on the street. Notice the ones who have smiles on their faces. Those folks are enjoying their walk; they are appreciating the scenery. There is no more profound advice than "stop and smell the roses."

Gratitude comes naturally to some people. They see the glass as half full. But most of us must cultivate that approach to life. We live in a culture where complaining is an art form and lack of appreciation a bad habit. (Lesowitz & Sammons) An "attitude of gratitude" will not only change your outlook and mood- it truly changes circumstances.

Sources:

Duesterhoeft, Cathy. *Live Well; Live Happy.* 2013

Lesowitz, Nina & Mary Beth Sammons. *Living Life as a Thank You. Viva Editions.* 2009